INTERVENTIONAL CARDIOLOGY CLINICS

www.interventional.theclinics.com

Editor-in-Chief

MARVIN H. ENG

Pulmonary Embolism Interventions

July 2023 • Volume 12 • Number 3

Editor

Vikas Aggarwal

ELSEVIER

1600 John F. Kennedy Boulevard ● Suite 1800 ● Philadelphia, Pennsylvania, 19103-2899

http://www.theclinics.com

INTERVENTIONAL CARDIOLOGY CLINICS Volume 12, Number 3
July 2023 ISSN 2211-7458, ISBN-13: 978-0-443-18207-5

Editor: Joanna Gascoine
Developmental Editor: Arlene B. Campos

© **2023 Elsevier Inc. All rights reserved.**

This periodical and the individual contributions contained in it are protected under copyright by Elsevier, and the following terms and conditions apply to their use:

Photocopying

Single photocopies of single articles may be made for personal use as allowed by national copyright laws. Permission of the Publisher and payment of a fee is required for all other photocopying, including multiple or systematic copying, copying for advertising or promotional purposes, resale, and all forms of document delivery. Special rates are available for educational institutions that wish to make photocopies for non-profit educational classroom use. For information on how to seek permission visit www.elsevier.com/permissions or call: (+44) 1865 843830 (UK)/(+1) 215 239 3804 (USA).

Derivative Works

Subscribers may reproduce tables of contents or prepare lists of articles including abstracts for internal circulation within their institutions. Permission of the Publisher is required for resale or distribution outside the institution. Permission of the Publisher is required for all other derivative works, including compilations and translations (please consult www.elsevier.com/permissions).

Electronic Storage or Usage

Permission of the Publisher is required to store or use electronically any material contained in this periodical, including any article or part of an article (please consult www.elsevier.com/permissions). Except as outlined above, no part of this publication may be reproduced, stored in a retrieval system or transmitted in any form or by any means, electronic, mechanical, photocopying, recording or otherwise, without prior written permission of the Publisher.

Notice

No responsibility is assumed by the Publisher for any injury and/or damage to persons or property as a matter of products liability, negligence or otherwise, or from any use or operation of any methods, products, instructions or ideas contained in the material herein. Because of rapid advances in the medical sciences, in particular, independent verification of diagnoses and drug dosages should be made.

Although all advertising material is expected to conform to ethical (medical) standards, inclusion in this publication does not constitute a guarantee or endorsement of the quality or value of such product or of the claims made of it by its manufacturer.

Interventional Cardiology Clinics (ISSN 2211-7458) is published quarterly by Elsevier Inc., 360 Park Avenue South, New York, NY 10010-1710. Months of issue are January, April, July, and October. Subscription prices are USD 217 per year for US individuals, USD 570 for US institutions, USD 100 per year for US students, USD 217 per year for Canadian individuals, USD 679 for Canadian institutions, USD 100 per year for Canadian students, USD 308 per year for international individuals, USD 679 for international institutions, and USD 150 per year for international students. To receive student/resident rate, orders must be accompanied by name of affiliated institution, date of term, and the *signature* of program/residency coordinator on institution letterhead. Orders will be billed at individual rate until proof of status is received. Foreign air speed delivery is included in all *Clinics* subscription prices. All prices are subject to change without notice. **POSTMASTER:** Send address changes to *Interventional Cardiology Clinics*, Elsevier Health Sciences Division, Subscription Customer Service, 3251 Riverport Lane, Maryland Heights, MO 63043. **Customer Service: Telephone:** 1-800-654-2452 (U.S. and Canada); **1-314-447-8871** (outside U.S. and Canada). **Fax:** 1-314-447-8029. **E-mail:** journalscustomerservice-usa@elsevier.com (for print support); journalsonlinesupport-usa@elsevier.com (for online support).

Reprints. For copies of 100 or more of articles in this publication, please contact the Commercial Reprints Department, Elsevier Inc., 360 Park Avenue South, New York, NY 10010-1710. Tel.: 212-633-3874; Fax: 212-633-3820; E-mail: reprints@elsevier.com.

Printed in the United States of America.

CONTRIBUTORS

CONSULTING EDITOR

MARVIN H. ENG, MD
Structural Heart Program Medical Director,
Structural Heart Disease Fellowship Director,
Director of Cardiovascular Quality,
Banner University Medical Center,
Phoenix, Arizona, USA

EDITOR

VIKAS AGGARWAL, MD, MPH
Co-director, Pulmonary Embolism Program,
Director of Venous and Pulmonary Vascular
Interventions, Interventional Cardiology and
Endovascular Interventions, Assistant
Professor of Clinical Medicine, Division of
Cardiology, Department of Internal Medicine,
University of Michigan Health System, Frankel
Cardiovascular Center, Section of Cardiology,
Department of Internal Medicine, Veterans
Affairs Medical Center, Ann Arbor, Michigan,
USA

AUTHORS

AHMAD A. ABDUL-AZIZ, MD
Inova Heart and Vascular Institute, Inova
Fairfax Medical Campus, Falls Church,
Virginia, USA

KOHTARO ABE, MD, PhD
Lecturer, Faculty of Cardiovascular Medicine,
Graduate School of Medical Sciences, Kyushu
University, Higashi-Ku, Fukuoka, Japan

VIKAS AGGARWAL, MD, MPH
Co-director, Pulmonary Embolism Program,
Director of Venous and Pulmonary Vascular
Interventions, Interventional Cardiology and
Endovascular Interventions, Assistant Professor
of Clinical Medicine, Division of Cardiology,
Department of Internal Medicine, University of
Michigan Health System, Frankel
Cardiovascular Center, Section of Cardiology,
Department of Internal Medicine, Veterans
Affairs Medical Center, Ann Arbor, Michigan,
USA

HUSEYIN EMRE ARMAN, DO
Department of Medicine, Indiana University
School of Medicine, Indianapolis, Indiana, USA

PUNIT ARORA, MD
Department of Internal Medicine, Loyola
University Medical Center, Maywood, Illinois,
USA

JU YOUNG BAE, MD
Section of Cardiovascular Medicine,
Department of Internal Medicine, Yale New
Haven Health Bridgeport Hospital,
Bridgeport, Connecticut, USA

YEVGENIY BRAILOVSKY, DO, MSc
Department of Advanced Heart Failure
and Transplantation, Thomas Jefferson
University Hospital, Philadelphia,
Pennsylvania, USA

SAURAV CHATTERJEE, MD
Department of Cardiology, Zucker School of
Medicine at Hofstra/Northwell, Hempstead,
New York, USA; Franciscan Health, Lafayette,
Indiana, USA

AMIR DARKI, MD, MSc
Department of Interventional Cardiology,
Associate Professor of Medicine, Cardiology,

Interventional Cardiologist, Loyola University Medical Center, Co-Director, Pulmonary Embolism Response Team, Maywood, Illinois, USA

PARTH V. DESAI, MD, MSc
Department of Interventional Cardiology, Loyola University Medical Center, Maywood, Illinois, USA

NAGA DHARMAVARAM, MD
Division of Cardiology, Department of Medicine, University of Wisconsin-Madison, Madison, Wisconsin, USA

AMIR ESMAEELI, MD
Division of Cardiology, Department of Medicine, University of Wisconsin-Madison, Madison, Wisconsin, USA

JAY GIRI, MD
Cardiovascular Medicine Division, Department of Medicine, Hospital of the University of Pennsylvania, Philadelphia, Pennsylvania, USA

GHAZALEH GOLDAR, MD
Cleveland Clinic Department of Cardiovascular Medicine, Heart, Vascular, and Thoracic Institute, Cleveland, Ohio, USA

JONATHAN W. HAFT, MD
Resident, Cardiothoracic Surgery, Professor of Cardiac Surgery, University of Michigan, Ann Arbor, Michigan, USA

KAZUYA HOSOKAWA, MD, PhD
Assistant Professor, Faculty of Cardiovascular Medicine, Graduate School of Medical Sciences, Kyushu University, Higashi-Ku, Fukuoka, Japan

SYED NABEEL HYDER, MD
Division of Cardiology, Department of Internal Medicine, University of Michigan, Ann Arbor, Michigan, USA

JULIA IOURINETS, BS
Stritch School of Medicine, Loyola University Chicago, Maywood, Illinois, USA

KURT JACOBSON, MD
Division of Cardiology, Department of Medicine, University of Wisconsin-Madison, Madison, Wisconsin, USA

NISHANT JAIN, MD
Department of Internal Medicine, University of Michigan, Ann Arbor, Michigan, USA

ANKUR KALRA, MD
Director, Interventional Services, New York Community Hospital, Brooklyn, New York, USA

KEVIN KHEDER, MD
Department of Interventional Cardiology, Loyola University Medical Center, Maywood, Illinois, USA

RICHARD A. KRASUSKI, MD
Professor of Medicine and Pediatrics, Division of Cardiology, Duke University Health System, Durham, North Carolina, USA

RAN LEE, MD
Cleveland Clinic Department of Cardiovascular Medicine, Heart, Vascular, and Thoracic Institute, Cleveland, Ohio, USA

ANAND REDDY MALIGIREDDY, MD
Division of Cardiology, Mayo Clinic, Scottsdale, Arizona, USA

KARTHIK MURUGIAH, MD
Assistant Professor of Medicine, Section of Cardiovascular Medicine, Department of Internal Medicine, Yale School of Medicine, Center for Outcomes Research and Evaluation, Yale New Haven Hospital, New Haven, Connecticut, USA

SIDNEY PERKINS, MSc
University of Michigan Medical School, Ann Arbor, Michigan, USA

KRISHNAN RAGHAVENDRAN, MD
Division of Acute Care Surgery, Department of Surgery, University of Michigan, Ann Arbor, Michigan, USA

FARHAN RAZA, MD
Division of Cardiology, Department of Medicine, University of Wisconsin-Madison, Madison, Wisconsin, USA

KENNETH ROSENFIELD, MD
Division of Cardiology, Department of Internal Medicine, Massachusetts General Hospital, Boston, Massachusetts, USA

MUHAMMAD ADIL SHEIKH, MD
Division of Cardiology, Department of Internal Medicine, Southern Illinois University, Springfield, Illinois, USA

SUPRIYA SHORE, MD, MSCS
University of Michigan Department of Internal Medicine, Ann Arbor, Michigan, USA

AARON A. SIFUENTES, MD
University of Michigan Department of Internal Medicine, Ann Arbor, Michigan, USA

PHANICHARAN SISTLA, MD
Department of Interventional Cardiology, Loyola University Medical Center, Maywood, Illinois, USA

MADATHILPARAMBIL V. SURESH, PhD
Division of Acute Care Surgery, Department of Surgery, University of Michigan, Ann Arbor, Michigan, USA

MANASI TANNU, MD, MPH
Division of Cardiology, Duke University Health System, Durham, North Carolina, USA

GABRIELLA VANAKEN, MD Candidate
University of Michigan School of Medicine, Ann Arbor, Michigan, USA

SCOTT H. VISOVATTI, MA, MD
Associate Professor, Department of Internal Medicine, Division of Cardiovascular Medicine, The Ohio State University, Davis Heart and Lung Research Institute, Columbus, Ohio, USA

YUZO YAMASAKI, MD, PhD
Assistant Professor, Department of Clinical Radiology, Graduate School of Medical Sciences, Kyushu University, Higashi-Ku, Fukuoka, Japan

GARDNER YOST, MD, MS
Resident, Cardiothoracic Surgery, University of Michigan, Ann Arbor, Michigan, USA

HARSHVARDHAN ZALA, MD, MSCR
Division of Cardiovascular Medicine, Department of Medicine, Indiana University School of Medicine, Indianapolis, Indiana, USA

CONTENTS

> Invasive or selective pulmonary angiography has historically been used as the gold standard diagnostic test for the evaluation of a wide array of pulmonary arterial conditions, most commonly pulmonary thromboembolic diseases. With the emergence of various noninvasive imaging modalities, the role of invasive pulmonary angiography is shifting to the assistance of advanced pharmacomechanical therapies for such conditions. Components of invasive pulmonary angiography methodology include optimal patient positioning, vascular access, catheter selections, angiographic positioning, contrast settings, and recognition of angiographic patterns of common thromboembolic and nonthromboembolic conditions. We review the pulmonary vascular anatomy, step-by-step performance, and interpretation of invasive pulmonary angiography.

> Venous thromboembolism is a common disorder encompassing both pulmonary embolism (PE) and deep vein thrombosis (DVT). In the United States, up to 2 million people are diagnosed with DVT and 600,000 with PE annually. The purpose of this review is to discuss the indications and evidence for catheter-directed thrombolysis versus catheter-based thrombectomy.

> Hemodynamically significant pulmonary embolism (PE) remains a widely prevalent, underdiagnosed condition associated with mortality rates as high as 30%. The main driver of poor outcomes is acute right ventricular failure that remains clinically challenging to diagnose and requires critical care management. Treatment of high-risk (or massive) acute PE has traditionally included systemic anticoagulation and thrombolysis. Mechanical circulatory support, including both percutaneous and surgical approaches, are emerging as treatment options for refractory shock due to acute right ventricular failure in the setting of high-risk acute pulmonary embolism.

> Acute pulmonary embolism (PE) is a common cause of death and morbidity in the United States and the prevalence of chronic thromboembolic pulmonary hypertension (CTEPH), a possible sequela of PE, has increased during the past decade. The mainstay treatment of CTEPH is open pulmonary endarterectomy, a procedure performed under hypothermic circulatory arrest, which entails endarterectomy of the branch, segmental and subsegmental pulmonary arteries. Acute PE may be similarly be treated with an open embolectomy in certain select circumstances.

Long-term exercise intolerance and functional limitations are common after an episode of acute pulmonary embolism (PE), despite 3 to 6 months of anticoagulation. These persistent symptoms are reported in more than half of the patients with acute PE and are referred as "post-PE syndrome." Although these functional limitations can occur from persistent pulmonary vascular occlusion or pulmonary vascular remodeling, significant deconditioning can be a major contributing factor. Herein, the authors review the role of exercise testing to elucidate the mechanisms of exercise limitations to guide next steps in management and exercise training for musculoskeletal deconditioning.

Chronic thromboembolic pulmonary hypertension (CTEPH) is a late complication of acute pulmonary thromboembolism owing to incomplete clot dissolution in pulmonary artery. Pulmonary endarterectomy is the first-line treatment for CTEPH. However, 40% of patients are not candidates for surgery because of distal lesions or age. Balloon pulmonary angioplasty (BPA), a catheter-based intervention, is increasingly being used worldwide for treating inoperable CTEPH. Previous BPA strategy had a major concern of reperfusion pulmonary edema as a complication. However, recent refined strategies promise safe and effective BPA. Five-year survival rate after BPA is 90% for inoperable CTEPH, comparable with that of operable CTEPH.

Pulmonary arterial hypertension (PAH) is a progressive, life-limiting disease. Despite significant medical progress over the last three decades, the prognosis of PAH remains poor. PAH is associated with sympathetic nervous system overstimulation and baroreceptor-mediated vasoconstriction, leading to pathologic pulmonary artery (PA) and right ventricular remodeling. PA denervation is a minimally-invasive intervention that ablates local sympathetic nerve fibers and baroreceptors to modulate pathologic vasoconstriction. Preliminary animal and clinical studies have shown improvements in short-term pulmonary hemodynamics and PA remodeling. However, future studies are needed to elucidate appropriate patient selection, timing of intervention, and long-term efficacy before integration into standard of care.

Center of excellence (COE) designations are generally used to identify programs with expertise in a specific area of medicine. Meeting criteria for a COE may result in advantages including improved clinical outcomes, marketing advantages, and improved financial performance. However, criteria for COE designations are highly variable, and they are granted by a wide variety of entities. The diagnosis and treatment of both acute pulmonary emboli and chronic thromboembolic pulmonary hypertension are disciplines that require multidisciplinary expertise, highly coordinated care, specialized technology and advanced skillsets gained through high patient volumes.

Venous thromboembolism (VTE) usually develops in the deep veins of the extremities. Pulmonary embolism (PE) is a type of VTE that is most commonly ($\sim$90%) caused by a thrombus that originates from the deep veins of the lower extremities. PE is the third most common cause of death after myocardial infarction and stroke. In this review, the authors investigate and discuss the risk stratification and definitions of different categories of PE and further explore the management of acute PE along with the types of catheter-based treatment options and their efficacy.

Balloon pulmonary angioplasty (BPA) was first described in 2001 and now has evolved into a class I indication for inoperable or residual chronic thromboembolic pulmonary hypertension. This review article aims to describe evidence from studies performed at various pulmonary hypertension (PH) centers across the globe, to better understand the role of BPA in chronic thromboembolic pulmonary disease with and without PH. Additionally, we hope to highlight innovations and the ever-changing safety and efficacy profile of BPA.

Many patients discharged after an acute pulmonary embolism (PE) admission have inconsistent outpatient follow-up and insufficient workup for chronic complications of PE. A structured outpatient care program is lacking for the different phenotypes of chronic PE, such as chronic thromboembolic disease, chronic thromboembolic pulmonary hypertension, and post-PE syndrome. A dedicated pulmonary embolism follow-up clinic and multi-disciplinary chronic PE team extends the organized, systematic care provided to PE patients via the inpatient PERT (Pulmonary Embolism Response Team) model into the outpatient setting. Such an initiative can standardize follow-up protocols after PE, limit unnecessary testing and ensure adequate management of chronic complications such as CTED, CTEPH, and the lesser defined phenotypes of post-PE syndrome. These clinics also have the potential to serve as platforms for clinical research in this rapidly evolving area.

Hypoxia-inducible factors (HIFs) are a family of nuclear transcription factors that serve as the master regulator of the adaptive response to hypoxia. In the lung, HIFs orchestrate multiple inflammatory pathways and signaling. They have been reported to have a major role in the initiation and progression of acute lung injury, chronic obstructive pulmonary disease, pulmonary fibrosis, and pulmonary hypertension. Although there seems to be a clear mechanistic role for both HIF 1α and 2α in pulmonary vascular diseases including PH, a successful translation into a definitive therapeutic modality has not been accomplished to date.

PULMONARY EMBOLISM INTERVENTIONS

FORTHCOMING ISSUES

October 2023
Multi-Modality Interventional Imaging
Thomas W. Smith, *Editor*

January 2024
Renal Disease and coronary, peripheral and structural interventions
Shweta Bansal, *Editor*

RECENT ISSUES

April 2023
Intracoronary Imaging and Its Use in Interventional Cardiology
Yasuhiro Honda, *Editor*

January 2023
Coronary Physiology in Contemporary Clinical Practice
Allen Jeremias, *Editor*

October 2022
Complex Coronary Interventions
Michael Lee, *Editor*

SERIES OF RELATED INTEREST

Cardiology Clinics
Cardiac Electrophysiology Clinics
Heart Failure Clinics

THE CLINICS ARE NOW AVAILABLE ONLINE!

Access your subscription at:
www.theclinics.com

FOREWORD

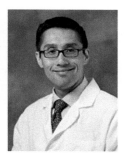

Marvin H. Eng, MD
Consulting Editor

We are pleased to introduce this issue of *Interventional Cardiology Clinics* that comprehensively covers transcatheter pulmonary interventions. From this issue, we can learn the state-of-the-art evolution of transcatheter pulmonary interventions from acute pulmonary embolism therapy to burgeoning therapies, such as pulmonary renal denervation. Fundamentals, such as pulmonary angiography and refamiliarization with vascular anatomy, are given due dedication, but focused discussion about developing the future of this interventional niche makes this a timely and well-thought-out issue. Special attention to preprocedural considerations, such as treatment of patients in cardiogenic shock, is discussed, and the controversies are explored. Just as importantly, detailed recommendations of postintervention care and rehabilitation complete the issue. Ultimately, just as we have "heart" teams, this issue describes the composition and function of a "lung" team.

This issue of *Interventional Cardiology Clinics* has been edited by Dr Vikas Aggrawal, a premier expert in pulmonary intervention. We congratulate Dr Aggrawal for assembling this complete treatise on the interventional aspects of treating pulmonary hypertension, acute pulmonary embolism, and building programs. Undoubtedly, the knowledge concentrated in this issue can serve as the blueprint for building centers of excellence and forging the future in pulmonary care.

Marvin H. Eng, MD
Structural Heart Program
Banner University Medical Center
1111 East McDowell Road
Phoenix, AZ 85006, USA

E-mail address:
engm@email.arizona.edu

Intervent Cardiol Clin 12 (2023) xi
https://doi.org/10.1016/j.iccl.2023.05.001
2211-7458/23/© 2023 Published by Elsevier Inc.

PREFACE

Toward a New Frontier in Acute and Chronic Pulmonary Embolism: Emerging Interventional Therapy Preeminence

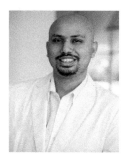

Vikas Aggarwal, MD, MPH
Editor

It is my pleasure and honor to introduce this latest issue of *Interventional Cardiology Clinics* dedicated to "Pulmonary Embolism Interventions." This issue highlights Pulmonary Embolism (PE), a rapidly evolving field within cardiovascular medicine at this time.

PE has been largely managed with anticoagulation alone for several decades, and advanced therapies were historically limited to extreme high-risk phenotypes. Over the past decade, PE care has seen a remarkable revolution in terms of care delivery as well as with the availability of new therapeutics.

This revolution has been led by the Pulmonary Embolism Response Team (PERT) framework that conceptualizes much needed multidisciplinary care for such patients. Originally conceived as a process improvement strategy for acutely ill patients with PE in the hospital, the PERT concept is now seeing adoption not only in the inpatient setting but also in the form of dedicated multidisciplinary Pulmonary Embolism Outpatient Clinics and in the management of chronic pulmonary thromboembolic disease.

The PERT phenomenon combined with the emergence of several catheter-based therapeutics in the form of thrombolysis/thrombectomy for acute disease and angioplasty for chronic disease has also reinvigorated interest in further study of established therapies, such as anticoagulation, systemic thrombolysis, open surgical approaches, and mechanical circulatory support for PE.

Together, multidisciplinary PE care and multiple medical, catheter, and open surgical treatment options are poised to positively impact PE-related mortality across phenotypes. In the same spirit, this issue of *Interventional Cardiology Clinics* brings to you an incredible, multidisciplinary group of experts in the field of pulmonary thromboembolism, who discuss all facets of this

Intervent Cardiol Clin 12 (2023) xiii–xiv
https://doi.org/10.1016/j.iccl.2023.03.001
2211-7458/23/© 2023 Published by Elsevier Inc.

incredibly complex disease process. We cover the past, present, and future of PE therapies, and present novel concepts for further discovery.

I want to thank the many individuals who helped with this effort, either directly or indirectly. From the incredible team at *Interventional Cardiology Clinics*, to the authors of the individual articles, to the members of our PE team at Michigan Medicine, to my family and friends, this issue is a culmination of all the support and all the hard work you have put into it. Thanks for your dedication to PE as a field, to the care of your patients as individuals, and to me personally as a friend and colleague. And, finally, to all the readers of this issue of *Interventional Cardiology Clinics*, thank you for allowing us to participate indirectly in the care of your patients.

Vikas Aggarwal, MD, MPH
Interventional Cardiology and
Endovascular Interventions
Division of Cardiology/
Department of Internal Medicine
University of Michigan Health System/
Frankel Cardiovascular Center
1500 East Medical Center Drive
Cardiovascular Center 2A181B, SPC 5869
Ann Arbor, MI 48109-5869, USA

E-mail address:
aggarwav@med.umich.edu

Invasive Pulmonary Angiogram Performance and Interpretation in the Diagnosis of Pulmonary Thromboembolic Disease

Ju Young Bae, MD[a], Karthik Murugiah, MD[b,c],*

KEYWORDS

- Chronic thromboembolic pulmonary hypertension • Interventional imaging
- Invasive pulmonary angiogram • Pulmonary thromboembolic disease

KEY POINTS

- Proper equipment, catheter position, contrast settings, and image acquisition technique can optimize pulmonary angiogram quality.
- Providing clear patient instruction during the procedure can improve angiographic image acquisition.
- Reviewing and complementing information from previous noninvasive imaging improves interpretation of pulmonary angiograms.

INTRODUCTION/HISTORY/DEFINITIONS/BACKGROUND

Invasive or selective pulmonary angiography, first described by Sasahara and colleagues[1] in 1964, was historically used as the gold standard diagnostic test for the evaluation of a wide array of congenital and acquired pulmonary arterial conditions, most commonly pulmonary thromboembolic diseases. However, with the emergence of various minimally invasive imaging modalities, such as computed tomographic pulmonary angiography, ventilation-perfusion lung scanning (V/Q scan), and magnetic resonance angiography, the role of invasive pulmonary angiography (IPA) is shifting largely to the assistance of advanced pharmacomechanical therapies for such conditions as chronic thromboembolic pulmonary hypertension (CTEPH), pulmonary arteriovenous malformations, pulmonary artery stenosis and aneurysms, and pulmonary artery neoplasms.[2] Understanding pulmonary vascular anatomy and the optimal pulmonary angiography technique is crucial for the invasive management of CTEPH. In this issue dedicated to pulmonary vascular interventions, we review the pulmonary arterial anatomy, procedural planning, patient positioning, and step-by-step performance of IPA, and interpretation of the most common thromboembolic conditions using IPA.

NATURE OF THE PROBLEM/DIAGNOSIS

With the proliferation of interventional therapies for pulmonary thrombotic and vascular conditions, training in and the understanding of IPA is valuable. This review describes in detail the best practices for this procedure and interpretation of findings.

---

[a] Section of Cardiovascular Medicine, Department of Internal Medicine, Yale New Haven Health Bridgeport Hospital, 267 Grant Street, Bridgeport, CT 06610, USA; [b] Section of Cardiovascular Medicine, Department of Internal Medicine, Yale University School of Medicine, New Haven, CT, USA; [c] Center for Outcomes Research and Evaluation, Yale New Haven Hospital, 195 Church Street, 6th Floor, New Haven, CT 06510, USA
* Corresponding author.
E-mail address: karthik.murugiah@yale.edu

Intervent Cardiol Clin 12 (2023) 299–307
https://doi.org/10.1016/j.iccl.2023.03.002
2211-7458/23/© 2023 Elsevier Inc. All rights reserved.

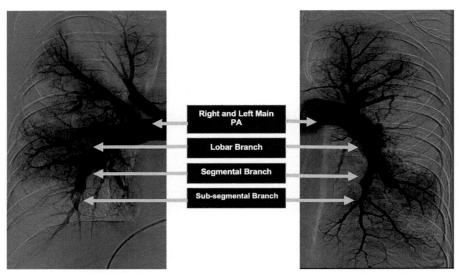

Fig. 1. Angiographic demonstration of pulmonary arterial circulation. PA, pulmonary artery.

DISCUSSION
Anatomy
Pulmonary arterial circulation
The pulmonary circulatory system is composed of the pulmonary arteries, pulmonary veins, and bronchial arteries. The main pulmonary artery (MPA) arises superiorly from the pulmonary annulus surrounding the base of the right ventricle (RV) coursing posteriorly and superiorly and then bifurcates into the right pulmonary artery (RPA) and left pulmonary artery (LPA) below the aortic arch to the left of the midline. The RPA and LPA divide into lobar branches and subsequently into segmental and subsegmental branches. These branches run in parallel to the segmental and subsegmental bronchi (**Fig. 1**).[3] Therefore, the segmental arteries are named according to the bronchopulmonary segment they perfuse.

Right pulmonary artery
The right upper lobe is supplied by the corresponding three segmental arteries (apical, A1; posterior, A2; anterior, A3), right middle lobe is supplied by two segmental arteries (lateral, A4; medial, A5), and right lower lobe by five segmental arteries (superior, A6; medial basal, A7; anterior basal, A8; lateral basal, A9; posterior basal, A10). The segmental arteries and their course in an anteroposterior and lateral view are shown in **Fig. 2**.

The RPA divides into two lobar branches, the truncus anterior (superior trunk) and the pars interlobaris (interlobar artery or inferior branch). The truncus anterior branches into two segmental

upper lobe arteries (A1 and A3). The A1 courses apically and the A3 courses anteriorly. The pars interlobaris continues toward the hilum first supplying a posterior coursing upper segmental artery (A2) and then two middle lobe arteries (A4 and A5). The middle lobe is an anterior structure and thus the A4 and A5 originate together anteriorly from the pars interlobaris and then the A4 courses laterally and the A5 medially. The pars interlobaris then courses inferiorly as the pars basalis and supplies the lower lobe through five segmental arteries. First the A6 originates, which supplies the superior segment of the lower lobe, which lies posterior to the middle lobe. The A6 divides into a medial and a lateral subsegmental branch. Subsequently, the anteromedial trunk and posterolateral trunk originate, which divide into A7/A8 and A9/A10 segmental arteries, respectively. The A7 and A8 are well separated in the frontal projection with the A7 coursing medially. The two trunks are well defined in the lateral projection.

Left pulmonary artery
The left upper lobe is supplied by four corresponding segmental arteries (apical-posterior, A1/A2; anterior, A3; superior lingular, A4; inferior lingular, A5), and the left lower lobe is supplied by four segmental arteries (superior, A6; anteromedial basal, A7/A8; lateral basal, A9; posterior basal, A10). The segmental arteries and their course in an anteroposterior and lateral view are shown in **Fig. 3**.

The LPA has a highly variable branching pattern. There is usually a larger artery supplying

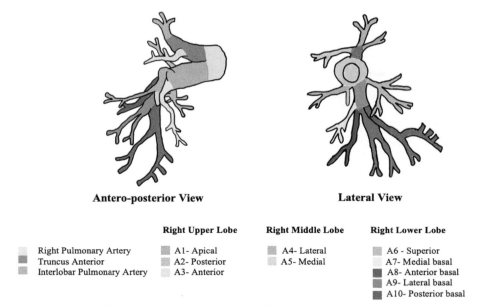

Antero-posterior View   **Lateral View**

	Right Upper Lobe	Right Middle Lobe	Right Lower Lobe
Right Pulmonary Artery	A1- Apical	A4- Lateral	A6 - Superior
Truncus Anterior	A2- Posterior	A5- Medial	A7- Medial basal
Interlobar Pulmonary Artery	A3- Anterior		A8- Anterior basal
			A9- Lateral basal
			A10- Posterior basal

Fig. 2. Anteroposterior and lateral representation of right pulmonary artery and segmental arteries.

the anterior segment of the upper lobe. The apical-posterior (A1/A2) branch courses apically and posteriorly. The A3 branch courses anteriorly and laterally. After this the lingular branches (A4 and A5) arise anteriorly and course laterally in a superior and inferior direction, respectively. There is a paucity of medial branches in the anterior areas of the left lung because of the heart. The first lower lobe branch is the A6, which courses posteriorly and has a medial and lateral

branch similar to that of the right side. The A7/A8 is a common segmental artery, which courses laterally. The A9 and A10 similar to the right side courses posteriorly.

Angiographic Technique
Preprocedure planning
Preprocedural assessment of patients includes a review of relevant medical history and allergies; electrocardiogram; and recent laboratory tests

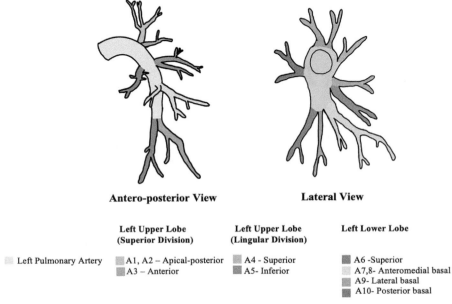

Antero-posterior View   **Lateral View**

	Left Upper Lobe (Superior Division)	Left Upper Lobe (Lingular Division)	Left Lower Lobe
Left Pulmonary Artery	A1, A2 – Apical-posterior	A4 - Superior	A6 -Superior
	A3 – Anterior	A5- Inferior	A7,8- Anteromedial basal
			A9- Lateral basal
			A10- Posterior basal

Fig. 3. Anteroposterior and lateral representation of left pulmonary artery and segmental arteries.

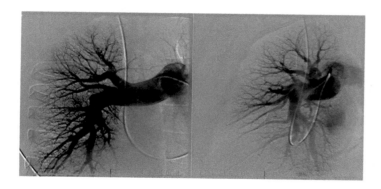

Fig. 4. Angiographic projections: frontal and lateral views of right pulmonary vasculature.

including hemoglobin, platelet count, renal function, coagulation parameters, and pregnancy screening.

Information regarding intracardiac devices, such as pacemakers, inferior vena cava (IVC) filters, and history of prior internal jugular (IJ) or femoral vein occlusive disease and superior vena cava or IVC stenoses should be obtained. Any prior investigations, such as transthoracic echocardiogram, computed tomographic pulmonary angiography, or V/Q scans need to be reviewed in detail to compare with the angiogram findings. Presence of a left bundle branch block should alert the provider to the possibility of complete heart block during the procedure. For a diagnostic pulmonary angiogram, interruption of therapeutic anticoagulation is preferred but not absolutely necessary. Most patients receive local or light conscious sedation during the procedure. Care should be taken to avoid deep sedation so that the patient can comply with breath holding during the procedure. Patients presenting for pulmonary angiograms often have tenuous hemodynamic status and need close hemodynamic and electrocardiographic monitoring.

Vascular access

The right IJ vein is the preferred approach because it serves as a smoother course for right heart catheterization using standard balloon-tipped, flow-directed catheters especially with a dilated right heart.[4] It also obviates a recumbent position after catheterization. In cases where the right IJ cannot be used, the left IJ or either common femoral vein is an alternate approach; the right femoral vein has a straighter course. Use of ultrasound guidance is paramount to exclude thrombosis of the access vein and facilitate safe access. A 7F or 8F catheter introducer sheath is preferable.

Equipment

Obtaining high-quality and safe angiograms requires the use of catheters with multiple-side hole, which can allow for power injections. Several options exist, such as the standard Berman catheter (Teleflex Inc, Wayne, PA); standard straight and curved pigtail shaped catheters; or specialized pulmonary catheters, such as the Grollman catheter (Cook Inc, Bloomington, IN). The standard Berman catheter (7F 90 cm, maximum flow rate 24 mL/s at 700

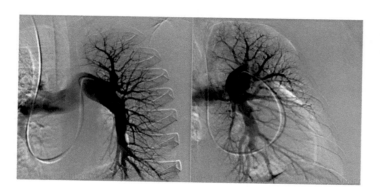

Fig. 5. Angiographic projections: frontal and lateral views of the left pulmonary vasculature.

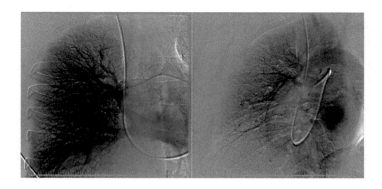

Fig. 6. Frontal and lateral angiograms of the right lung showing the levophase.

psi) is a balloon-tipped, end-capped pressure-rated catheter that facilitates easy flow-directed advancement from the right heart into the pulmonary artery.[4] The presence of an end cap provides protection of distal pulmonary vasculature from iatrogenic damage particularly during high-pressure contrast injections. Similarly, a high-flow straight or angled (preferable) pigtail is used. The Grollman catheter (6.7F 100 cm, maximum flow rate 27 mL/s at 765 psi) is another alternative, which has a 90° curve 3 cm proximal to the pigtail curve. End-hole Swan Ganz catheters should be avoided because they are not compatible with high-pressure injections.

Approach
Catheter position
The standard Berman catheter balloon is advanced from the right IJ similar to "floating" a Swan Ganz catheter. The balloon is inflated in the superior vena cava and when advanced the catheter should traverse the RV with ease and preferentially reach the RPA. When approaching from the femoral vein the balloon is inflated in the common iliac vein. Clockwise rotation of the catheter as it traverses the tricuspid valve assists in advancement to the pulmonary artery. Deep inspiration may facilitate catheter entry into the MPA. Alternatively, a loop is formed in the RA by curving the tip of the catheter against the lateral right atrial wall or by engaging in the hepatic vein ostium. This maneuver is helpful with a dilated RV. Catheter advancement should be done under continuous pressure wave monitoring. For instance, the catheter can enter the coronary sinus (CS) when advancing from the IJ or enter the left atrium via a patent foramen ovale or atrial septal defect. The absence of a transition to RV tracing should alert the operator. A hand injection of contrast can also confirm the catheter path.

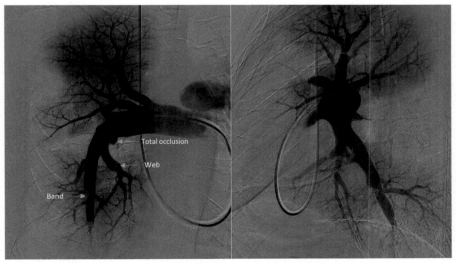

Fig. 7. Frontal and lateral angiograms of the right lung in a patient with CTEPH showing common lesion morphologies.

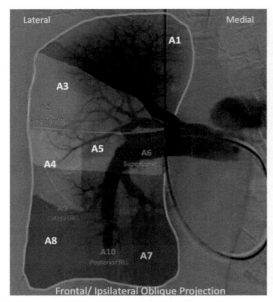
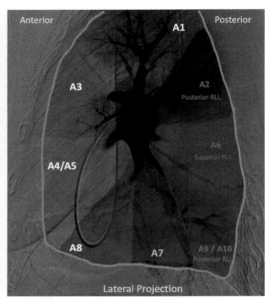

Fig. 8. Perfusion zones of the right lung in anteroposterior and lateral views. RLL, right lower lobe; RUL, right upper lobe.

The curved pigtail catheter or the Grollman catheter is advanced over wire until the IVC and then advanced without wire across the tricuspid valve. A counterclockwise rotation helps direct it toward the MPA. In challenging situations, the pulmonary artery is catheterized using a conventional balloon flotation catheter and exchanged for a pigtail catheter overwire. In most catheterizations the catheter preferentially enters the RPA. To cannulate the LPA, in

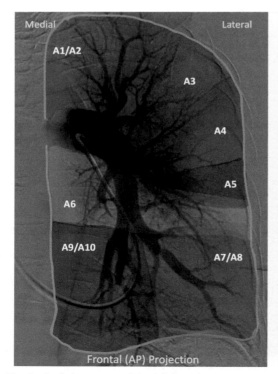
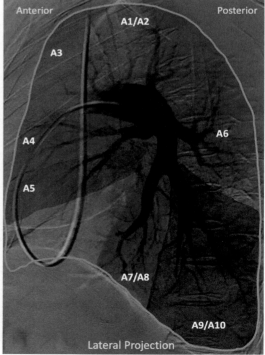

Fig. 9. Perfusion zones of the left lung in anteroposterior and lateral views.

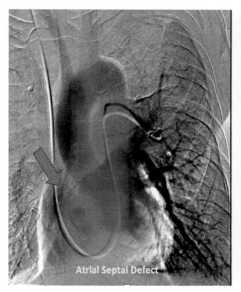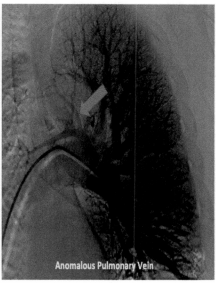

Atrial Septal Defect

Anomalous Pulmonary Vein

Fig. 10. Angiographic examples of nonthromboembolic pulmonary artery diseases.

case of a pigtail-shaped catheter, it is withdrawn into the MPA and redirected in a superior direction to enter the LPA. If unable to, the shaft of the pigtail in the MPA is stiffened using the proximal end of a 0.035 wire to allow cannulation of the LPA. A similar maneuver is used with the Berman catheter. Once the Berman catheter is in position the balloon is taken down in preparation for the angiogram.

To image the RPA and branches the angiographic catheter should be positioned beyond the origin of the truncus arteriosus and into the interlobar artery. The catheter in this position has reduced recoil. The middle and lower lobes are imaged first followed quickly by the refluxing contrast opacifying the upper lobe. To image the LPA and branches the catheter is positioned beyond the point where the LPA begins to course inferiorly. In either lung the catheter in position should not have excessive motion with the cardiac cycle in which case the catheter is advanced a few centimeters. However, care should be taken that the catheter is not immobile, which may suggest engagement into a clot/obstruction or a deep position of the catheter, in which case the catheter is withdrawn a few centimeters. Furthermore, the position of the catheter should be optimized to avoid contrast spillover to the contralateral lung, which can compromise image quality, especially for lateral projections.

Patient position

The patient should preferably be in a supine position with arms raised above shoulder level with

hands clasped behind head. This is especially important for patients with high body mass index or for any patient if lateral (90°) projections are obtained. It is important to ensure that the patient is comfortable in this position and able to perform an adequate breath hold for imaging, which is essential for optimal angiography quality. An evaluation of the breath hold should be conducted under fluoroscopy before obtaining digital subtraction angiography (DSA) images. In addition, the catheter's position with deep inspiration can also be observed and adjustments made. If the patient is unable to hold their breath, then a cine-angiography should be obtained instead of DSA, which although suboptimal provides interpretable information.

Contrast injection

Contrast is diluted with saline at a 3:1 dilution to reduce contrast amount. Contrast is delivered typically through a power injector at 18 to 20 mL/s for 2.0 seconds at a minimum of 600 psi. The flow rate and volume should be reduced in cases of severely reduced cardiac output or extensive CTEPH burden to 15 mL/s for 2 seconds. For significant pulmonary hypertension but moderate CTEPH disease burden, reduce flow rate to 15 mL/s to minimize hemodynamic consequences, but the duration can be extended to 2.5 seconds so the pulmonary vasculature is filled adequately. A test injection with 5 to 10 mL can allow the operator to gauge the extent of proximal CTEPH and antegrade flow through the vessel and calibrate the contrast settings. Ang and colleagues[4] have

Table 1
Summary of angiographic patterns of nonthromboembolic pulmonary artery diseases on pulmonary angiograms

Disease Process	Angiographic Pattern
Main pulmonary artery stenosis	Pulmonary artery narrowing; pressure gradient on catheterization
Pulmonary artery aneurysm	Focal saccular or fusiform pulmonary arterial dilation with a wide neck
Pulmonary arteritis	Distal pulmonary artery stenoses or occlusions; can mimic CTEPH
Pulmonary artery neoplasms	Localized stenosis with irregular margins; can mimic CTEPH
Pulmonary artery agenesis	Absence of the right or left pulmonary artery with an intact main pulmonary artery
Pulmonary artery sling	Origin of the left pulmonary artery from the right pulmonary artery, coursing between the trachea and esophagus
Patent ductus arteriosus	Patent communication between descending aorta and pulmonary artery; can be seen as negative contrast but seen better on aortograms
Pulmonary arteriovenous malformation and fistula	Abnormal direct communication between the branches of the pulmonary artery and vein in such conditions as hereditary hemorrhagic telangiectasia
Atrial septal defect	Communication visualized between left and right atrium during levophase
Partial anomalous pulmonary venous connection	One or more pulmonary veins draining into the right atrium during levophase
Pulmonary vein stenosis	Stenosis of one or more pulmonary veins as they drain into the left atrium in the levophase

suggested contrast settings based on body size, cardiac index, and disease severity.

Angiographic projections
Angiograms are obtained using DSA. Two orthogonal projections should be obtained for comprehensive interpretation of all pulmonary segmental anatomy. We suggest for the right lung right anterior oblique (RAO) 20° to 45° (frontal projection) and left anterior oblique (LAO) 30° to 45° (lateral projection) (Fig. 4) and for the left lung LAO 20° to 45° (frontal projection) and RAO 30° to 45° (lateral projection). Alternatively, for the right lung, a straight anteroposterior and LAO 90° is used (Fig. 5).[4] A straight projection should not be taken of the left lung to avoid overlap from the mediastinum. Optimization of views should be based on individual anatomy. Imaging should be continued beyond arterial system opacification and until the pulmonary venous system fills (levophase), because this is important for a complete assessment (Fig. 6). Collimate in both axes to maximize the lung fields. Biplane angiography can

help greatly reduce contrast volume and radiation exposure; however, it may not be available at many centers. Digital processing settings should be optimized for optimal brightness and contrast and to reduce artifact. Different angiographic systems may have preset optimized settings for pulmonary angiograms.

Imaging
Angiographic patterns of chronic thromboembolic pulmonary hypertension
Angiography findings in CTEPH can involve the MPA and lobar arteries (proximal disease) or involve the segmental and subsegmental arteries (distal disease). Proximal disease imaging findings can also include filling defects, which suggest acute emboli, seen in CTEPH patients. The remainder of the lesions, similar to that seen in distal disease, are bands or ringlike stenoses, weblike lesions, subtotal occlusions, and total occlusions/pouch defects (Fig. 7).[5,6]

An understanding of the perfusion zones and respective segmental arteries (Figs. 8 and 9) is helpful to define the distribution of disease pathology and identify involved vessels to assist in planning catheter-based interventions.[6] To avoid missing total occlusions careful counting of major vessels is recommended, but natural variation in anatomy can complicate vessel origin identification.[4] It is often helpful to look at the distal lung perfusion on the angiograms and in the areas with poor perfusion follow backward centrally to identify lesions. It is critical to obtain imaging until the levophase. Reduced venous return in a particular segmental territory raises the suspicion of a corresponding segmental arterial stenosis. Sometimes weblike lesions are not clearly apparent on a nonselective angiogram and the venous return helps indirectly identify these lesions. It is also important to complement the angiogram with CTA and V/Q scan information. V/Q scans typically report the areas with reduced perfusion based on involved broncho-pulmonary segments.

Selective angiograms of segmental arteries taken during balloon pulmonary angioplasty demonstrate the presence and characteristics of CTEPH lesions with greater definition. However, these are typically obtained after the decision for balloon pulmonary angioplasty is made. In later articles in this issue selective angiograms are discussed. A high-quality nonselective pulmonary angiogram following the previously mentioned suggestions is sufficient in most cases to make the diagnosis and assess candidacy for invasive therapies.

Angiographic patterns of nonthromboembolic pulmonary artery diseases

Although this angiogram review is focused on imaging in CTEPH, in practice patients may present with undifferentiated dyspnea and no prior pulmonary vascular diagnoses. Thus, it remains important to be able to identify on pulmonary angiography patterns of nonthromboembolic pulmonary artery disease (**Fig. 10, Table 1**). Other pulmonary arterial conditions that are visible on coronary and not pulmonary arteriograms include coronary artery to pulmonary artery fistulae and anomalous coronaries originating from pulmonary artery.

SUMMARY

Invasive angiography remains a valuable technique in the diagnosis and management of numerous pulmonary thromboembolic diseases. Components of IPA methodology include optimal patient positioning, vascular access, catheter selections, angiographic positioning, contrast settings, and recognition of angiographic patterns of common thromboembolic and nonthromboembolic conditions.

CLINICS CARE POINTS

- Proper equipment, catheter position, contrast settings, and image acquisition technique can optimize pulmonary angiogram quality.
- Providing clear patient instruction during the procedure can improve angiographic image acquisition.
- Reviewing and complementing information from previous noninvasive imaging improves interpretation of pulmonary angiograms.

DISCLOSURES

Dr K. Murugiah received support from the National Heart, Lung, and Blood Institute, United States of the National Institutes of Health (under award K08HL157727), United States.

REFERENCES

1. Sasahara AA, Stein M, Simon M, et al. Pulmonary angiography in the diagnosis of thromboembolic disease. N Engl J Med 1964;270:1075–81.
2. Kandathil A, Chamarthy M. Pulmonary vascular anatomy & anatomical variants. Cardiovasc Diagn Ther 2018;8:201–7.
3. Patel N, Hyder S, Michaud E, et al. Interventional imaging roadmap to successful balloon pulmonary angioplasty for chronic thromboembolic pulmonary hypertension. JSCAI 2022;1:6.
4. Ang L, McDivit Mizzell A, Daniels LB, et al. Optimal technique for performing invasive pulmonary angiography for chronic thromboembolic pulmonary disease. J Invasive Cardiol 2019;31:E211–9.
5. Kawakami T, Ogawa A, Miyaji K, et al. Novel angiographic classification of each vascular lesion in chronic thromboembolic pulmonary hypertension based on selective angiogram and results of balloon pulmonary angioplasty. Circ Cardiovasc Interv 2016;9.
6. Aggarwal Vikas, Vladimir Lakhter. "How to interpret pulmonary angiogram." SCAI, 2021, Available at: https://scai.org/how-interpret-pulmonary-angiogram. Accessed November 19, 2022.

Catheter-Directed Thrombolysis or Catheter-Based Thrombectomy in Acute Pulmonary Embolism
Horses for Courses

Phanicharan Sistla, MD[a], Kevin Kheder, MD[a],
Julia Iourinets, BS[b], Punit Arora, MD[c],
Parth V. Desai, MD, MSc[a], Yevgeniy Brailovsky, DO, MSc[d],
Amir Darki, MD, MSc[a,e,*]

KEYWORDS

- Venous thromboembolism • Pulmonary embolism • Catheter-directed thrombolysis
- Catheter-based thrombectomy

KEY POINTS

- Venous thromboembolism is a heterogenous disorder whose presentation varies widely between asymptomatic and those at high risk for PE-related mortality.
- Patients at high risk for decompensation are risk-stratified by a combination of clinical, laboratory biomarkers (brain natriuretic peptide, troponin), imaging (computed tomography, ventilation-perfusion scan, and echo), and residual clot burden.
- A subset of PE patients at high risk for decompensation and death are candidates for two broad categories of endovascular intervention: catheter-directed thrombolysis (CDT) and catheter-based thrombectomy (CBT).
- CDT involves the direct infusion of thrombolytic agents into the clot via 4-6 Fr multi-hole catheters. The addition of ultrasound has the potential to increase fragmentation and enhance thrombolysis.
- CBT involves the advancement of a large-bore aspiration guide catheter to engage, disrupt, and extract the clot.

INTRODUCTION

Venous thromboembolism (VTE) is a common disorder encompassing both pulmonary embolism (PE) and deep vein thrombosis (DVT). In the United States, up to 2 million people are diagnosed with DVT and 600,000 with PE annually.[1] The reported incidence of PE has risen significantly over the past two decades due to a myriad of factors including an aging population, wider

Funding: No specific funding was associated with this research.
[a] Department of Interventional Cardiology, Loyola University Medical Center, 2160 South First Avenue, Maywood, IL 60153, USA; [b] Stritch School of Medicine, Loyola University Chicago, 2160 South First Avenue, Maywood, IL 60153, USA; [c] Department of Internal Medicine, Loyola University Medical Center, 2160 South First Avenue, Maywood, IL 60153, USA; [d] Department of Advanced Heart Failure and Transplantation, Thomas Jefferson University Hospital, 925 Chestnut Street, Philadelphia, PA 19107, USA; [e] Cardiology, Loyola University Medical Center, Pulmonary Embolism Response Team
* Corresponding author. Cardiology, Loyola University Medical Center, Pulmonary Embolism Response Team, 2160 South First Avenue, Maywood, IL 60153, USA
E-mail address: adarki@lumc.edu

Intervent Cardiol Clin 12 (2023) 309–321
https://doi.org/10.1016/j.iccl.2023.03.003
2211-7458/23/

use of imaging techniques,[2,3] and improved diagnostic algorithms providing a higher degree of specificity and sensitivity even for subclinical PE.[4] Despite advancements in detection and intervention, VTE remains the third most common cause of cardiovascular deaths in the United States, with approximately 30% of all PE patients presenting with sudden death from acute right ventricular (RV) failure or dying within a year of diagnosis.[5–7] The mainstay of treatment of PE has been systemic anticoagulation. More recently, there has been a rapid development of endovascular techniques to treat high-risk PE at risk of decompensation. The purpose of this review is to discuss the indications and evidence for catheter-directed thrombolysis (CDT) versus catheter-based thrombectomy (CBT) (Fig. 1).

PULMONARY EMBOLISM BACKGROUND
Clinical Presentation and Diagnostic Testing
Clinical presentation of PE can vary depending on the size of the embolus and cardiopulmonary status, ranging from asymptomatic to obstructive shock and sudden death. Typically, patients present with acute-onset dyspnea, cough, and pleuritic chest pain, often accompanied by clinical signs of tachypnea and hypoxia. A significant subset (about 4%–22%) of patients with PE will present with syncope.[8] The mechanisms underlying syncope in PE focus on factors that cause cerebral hypoperfusion, such as RV failure leading to decreased cardiac output, development of bradyarrhythmias, and vasovagal component with hypotension.[9] Patients with PE who present with syncope often have a larger clot burden that involves the main pulmonary or lobar arteries, decreased hemodynamic reserve,[10,11] and comprise approximately 30% of fatal PE cases. This warrants serious consideration of PE in the primary differential diagnosis for syncope, especially if there is no alternative explanation.[8,12,13]

Severity Classification
The American College of Chest Physicians and European Society of Cardiology (ESC) have outlined a classification system of PE severity based on short-term (30-day or in-hospital) mortality risk defined by the presence of shock, RV dysfunction, and integration of patient clinical status, laboratory markers of RV ischemia and strain, and comorbidities with risk stratification scores (ie, Simplified Pulmonary Embolism Severity Index [sPESI]). The *American Heart Association* (AHA) classifies PE into low-risk, submassive, and massive categories. The ESC classifies PE into low-risk, intermediate low/ high, and massive PE (Table 1).

Risk Stratification and Indications for Escalation of Therapy
After a timely diagnosis of acute pulmonary embolism (APE), risk stratification becomes critical, particularly in informing steps in escalation of care, admission to the intensive care unit (ICU), administration of thrombolytics, and performance of invasive procedures.

Although both the ESC and AHA guidelines are in agreement for systemic anticoagulation and an opportunity for early discharge in low-risk patients,[14] intermediate and massive PE frequently pose a more complicated diagnostic scenario.[15,16] Although less than 5% of patients present with massive PE (defined as systolic blood pressure [SBP] <90 mm Hg or a decrease in SBP > 40 mm Hg, new vasopressor requirements, or PE-associated shock), mortality remains high at over 30%, and thus they are candidates for immediate reperfusion therapy.[15,16] In the only randomized controlled thrombolysis trial, those with massive PE who were randomized to streptokinase improved within an hour of treatment, while those who received heparin alone progressed into cardiogenic shock and died, resulting in early termination of the trial after only four patients.[17] In those high-risk patients whose bleeding risk is also elevated, or if patients remain unstable despite systemic fibrinolysis, CBT, or surgical pulmonary embolectomy (SPE) should be considered.[15,16]

In patients with intermediate-risk or submassive PE, accurate prognostication of risk for decompensation is challenging. Given the low positive predictive value (20%) of PESI and sPESI, decisions to escalate therapy for those at high risk of early decompensation or mortality should be based on more granular information beyond current scoring systems. In such patients, factors such as biomarkers, proximal clot burden, RV/ left ventricle (LV) ratio, and RV hemodynamics on echo and computed tomography angiography (CTA) can help provide direction at high risk for deterioration (Fig. 2).

Laboratory biomarkers of brain natriuretic peptide (BNP), NT-proBNP, troponin, and lactate can help indicate RV strain, dilation, and myocardial ischemia to stratify normotensive patients with APE, as they are independent risk factors for short-term mortality and RV strain. A meta-analysis demonstrated that elevated BNP and NT-proBNP levels were associated with a higher risk of short-term death,

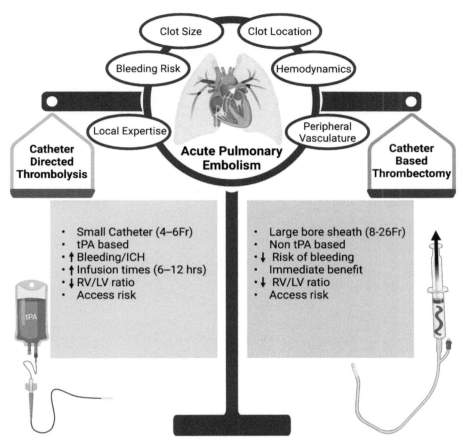

Fig. 1. Benefits and limitations of catheter-directed thrombolysis versus catheter-based thrombectomy. (Created with Biorender.com.)

Table 1
Classification of pulmonary embolism severity adapted from European Society of Cardiology and American Heart Association Guidelines

		Risk Indicators			
	Mortality Risk	Hemodynamic Instability	Imaging Evidence of RV Dysfunction	Elevation of Biomakers	Risk Stratification Score (PESI Class III-V or sPESI ≥1)
ESC	High	+	+	+	+
	Intermediate high	-	+	+	+
	Intermediate low	-	Either one +, or both -		+
	Low	-	-	-	-
AHA (2011)	Massive	+			
	Submassive	-	Either one +		
	Low	-	-	-	

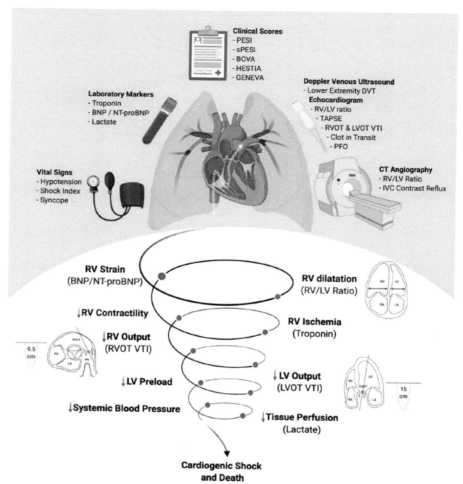

Fig. 2. Factors associated with decompensation and death in acute pulmonary embolism. (Created with Biorender. com.)

though there was low specificity to predict death.[18] In normotensive patients with PE, increased troponin levels were also associated with short-term mortality (OR 4.80, $P<.05$), however, like other biomarkers, elevated troponin cannot be used alone to determine the next steps as it only mildly improved diagnostic accuracy with a positive likelihood ratio of 2.13 and negative likelihood ratio of 0.51.[18] Elevated plasma lactate greater than 2 mmol/L, which can indicate decreased tissue perfusion in PE-related obstructive physiology, has been associated with an increased risk of all-cause death (HR 11.67) independent of shock, hypotension, RV dysfunction, or troponinemia.[19]

Although CTA is a gold standard for diagnosing APE, this readily available modality also helps stratify patients with increased risk of early mortality through assessment of RV functionality.

RV dysfunction, as measured by an RV/LV ratio > 0.9 in a meta-analysis, leads to an increase in all-cause (OR 2.5, $P<.0001$) and PE-related (OR 5.0, $P<.0001$) mortality.[18]

Echocardiography can similarly provide information on RV hemodynamics. An RV/LV ratio >0.9 has been shown to be an independent risk factor for in-hospital mortality (OR 2.66, $P =.01$).[20] As the RV dilates in acute pressure overload, it can no longer dilate to augment preload. This decreases RV and thus LV stroke volume which can be estimated by right ventricular outflow tract (RVOT) velocity time integral (VTI) and left ventricular outflow tract (LVOT) VTI, respectively. Reduced RVOT VTI was found to be a significant predictor of low cardiac index (CI). Specifically, RVOT VTI <10 cm and LVOT VTI <15 cm in intermediate-high-risk patients were linked to increased mortality.[18] The "60-60" sign, a measurement of estimated PA pressure < 60 mm Hg and an RVOT acceleration time < 60 milliseconds, identifies RV–PA uncoupling seen in APE physiology and is linked to an increase in mortality.[21] In intermediate-risk patients, tricuspid annular plane systolic excursion (TAPSE) < 16 mm was found to be an independent predictor of PE-specific mortality and reductions of TAPSE were linked with a need for thrombolysis, though positive predictive values were poor (20.9%).[18]

Right-heart thrombi and concomitant lower extremity DVT are additional sources of secondary emboli which may lead to increased morbidity and mortality.[18] The clot in transit, defined as a free-floating thrombus within the right atrium (RA) or RV, was associated with a higher risk of short-term all-cause mortality.[18]

In summary, early risk stratification is crucial in intermediate and high-risk PE. Although no one marker or imaging can adequately predict patients at risk of early mortality or deterioration, a combination of biomarkers, CT, and echo findings will help identify patients at high risk for decompensation and need for escalation.

ENDOVASCULAR THERAPIES FOR ACUTE PULMONARY EMBOLISM

The impetus for catheter-based treatment of intermediate and high-risk PE patients was the desire to reduce the risk of bleeding including intracranial hemorrhage (PIETHO). Broadly, there are two strategies within catheter-based therapies: CDT and CBT. Factors that help determine the best strategy include thrombus burden and location, bleeding risk, device availability, and operator experience (Table 2).

CATHETER-DIRECTED THROMBOLYSIS

CDT involves the placement of a catheter via the internal jugular (IJ) or femoral vein (FV) into the PA directly into the thrombus with an infusion of a thrombolytic agent to enhance clot dissolution. The goal of CDT is to produce superior efficacy to systemic thrombolysis with a significantly reduced dose, thus mitigating bleeding risk.

The number of infusion catheters and the dosing of tissue plasminogen activator (tPA) varies, with typical protocols ranging between 6 and 24 mg over 12 to 24 hours (ie, 1 mg/hour per lung for 6–12 hours).[22,23] Catheter placement into one or both PAs depends on unilateral or bilateral lung involvement and it is percutaneously placed under fluoroscopic guidance. Two

commonly used multi-side hole catheters are Uni-Fuse (Angiodynamics Inc, Latham, NY) and Cragg-McNamara (Medtronic, Minneapolis, MN). Catheter sizes range from 4- to 5-Fr with infusion lengths of 10 cm. Alternatively, the Eko-Sonic (EKOS) endovascular system (Boston Scientific Corp, Marlborough, MA) contains two lumens—one that emits ultrasound energy and the other to deliver thrombolytic therapy. Ultrasound-assisted thrombolysis (USAT) using high-intensity ultrasound energy is postulated to disrupt fibrin fibers, thus increasing the surface area available for tPA-enhancing thrombolysis.[24] Two prospective trials of USAT have been performed: ULTIMA and SEATTLE II.

In ULTIMA, 59 patients with intermediate-risk PE were randomized to USAT followed by IV heparin or IV heparin alone. The primary endpoint was the difference in RV/LV ratio from baseline to 24 hours, obtained from the echocardiographic apical 4-chamber view. At 24 hours, significant improvement in the primary endpoint was observed in the USAT group compared with the conventional anticoagulation group (mean change in RV/LV ratio -0.30 ± 0.019 vs -0.03 ± 0.016; $P<.001$). Additionally, a significant reduction in the RA/RV pressure gradient on an echocardiogram, a surrogate for PA pressure, was observed in favor of USAT (mean reduction 9.8 ± 9.9 vs 0.3 ± 10.9 mm Hg; $P =.03$). At 90 days, however, there was no difference in mortality or major bleeding events in either group.[22]

SEATTLE II was a prospective, single-arm study that enrolled 150 patients with intermediate-high risk (n = 119) or massive PE (n = 31) to evaluate the safety and efficacy of USAT. A notable difference from ULTIMA is that massive PE patients were included in this study. Two primary endpoints: efficacy outcome (change in RV/LV ratio from baseline at 48 hours assessed by CT) and safety outcome (major bleeding complications within 72 hours defined by global utilization of streptokinase and tPA for occluded arteries [GUSTO] moderate or severe) were analyzed. Secondary efficacy outcomes were changes in invasive PA pressure measurement and in modified Miller angiographic obstruction index score at 48 hours. The modified Miller index score quantifies the extent of thrombus in each PA and their segments by CT, with a maximal score of 40 corresponding with occlusion of all PA segments.[25] The total dose of tPA was 24 mg, regardless of unilateral or bilateral catheter placement. At 48 hours, USAT showed a significant reduction in RV/LV ratio (1.55 vs 1.13), mean PA pressure

Table 2
Devices used for endovascular interventions in pulmonary embolism

Device	Mechanism	Catheter Size	Technical Consideration
Uni-fuse	SCDT	4- to 5-Fr	• FDA-approved for peripheral vasculature without specific indication for PE • IJ or FV access • Low cost
Cragg-McNamara	SCDT	4- to 5-Fr	• FDA-approved for peripheral vasculature without specific indication for PE • IJ or femoral vein access • Low cost
EkoSonic (EKOS)	USAT	5-Fr	• FDA-approved for PE • IJ or FV access
Bashir (BEC)	PM-CDT	7-Fr	• Pending FDA approval for PE (RESCUE trial) • FV or IJ access
AngioVac	Veno-veno bypass	26-Fr inflow cannula, 16–20-Fr outflow cannula	• Perfusion team needed
Inari Flow Triever	Aspiration of clot and mechanical retrieval with mitinol disks	16-, 20-, or 24-Fr	• Blood loss (large-bore aspiration) • FlowSaver • FDA-approved
Penumbra Indigo	Mechanical aspiration of clot	8- or 12-Fr	• Indigo Lightning technology • Blood loss (large-bore aspiration) • FDA-approved
AngioJet	Rheolytic thrombectomy	8-Fr	• Hypotension, bradycardia • Black box warming

(51.4 vs 37.5 mm Hg), and mean modified Miller score (mean difference, -6.6).[23] There was one major bleeding event that was a GUSTO severe hemorrhage (access site hematoma requiring vasopressor support), the remaining bleeding events (94%) were moderate.[23] These results ultimately led to the Food and Drug Administration (FDA) approval of the EKOS catheter in 2014 for the treatment of APE (Fig. 3).

As the trend for CDT continues to increase, standardized tPA dosing algorithms and protocols will be crucial to ensure adequate thrombolysis while minimizing bleeding risk.[26] Although multiple studies have validated the safety and effectiveness of CDT therapy in APE, few trials have studied differences in dosing protocols. To address this need, the OPTALYSE-PE trial was designed to optimize USAT tPA dose and infusion duration;[27] 101 patients with acute intermediate-high risk PE were randomized to

one of four tPA dosing cohorts: 4 mg/lung over 2 hours, 4 mg/lung over 4 hours, 6 mg/lung over 6 hours, and 12 mg/lung over 6 hours evaluating the primary efficacy endpoint of RV/LV ratio by CT. The primary safety outcome was frequency of major bleeding within 72 hours by International Society on Thrombosis and Hemostasis criteria. A notable secondary endpoint was embolic burden by the modified Miller score on CT 48 hours after initiation of USAT. Each regimen improved RV/LV ratio and modified the Miller score compared with baseline, with an overall major bleeding rate of 4% and one intracranial hemorrhage in a patient given 4 mg/lung over 4 hours. Outcomes at 1 year showed sustained RV/LV recovery and improved quality of life. Although further studies are needed to evaluate different dosing strategies as compared with conservative management with anticoagulation, this trial demonstrated

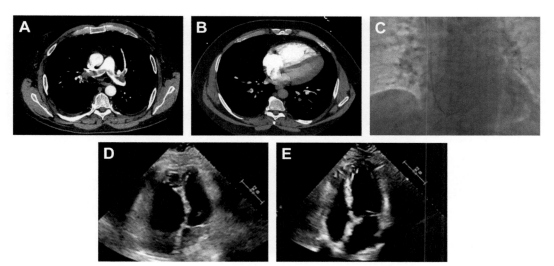

Fig. 3. (Case 1). (A) 76 year-old female presenting with acute-onset shortness of breath and found to have a large saddle PE with extensive bilateral clot burden. (B) CT with significant RV enlargement with interventricular septal flattening. (C) Bilateral EKOS catheters placed in right and left PA from a right IJ approach. (D) Echocardiogram with significant RV dilation in the apical-4 chamber view. (E) Echocardiogram apical-4 chamber with recovery of RV at 6 week follow-up following treatment with EKOS.

that lower doses and shorter infusions of thrombolytic therapy are safe and effective in acute submassive PE.

The EkoSonic EKOS Endovascular System combines an ultrasound core with the catheter and is currently the only ultrasound catheter approved by the FDA for the treatment of APE. The estimated cost is $14,500 for the control unit and $2295 for each individual infusion catheter.

This is a roughly 10-fold increase in cost compared with standard multi-hole infusion catheters. To date, multiple studies have failed to detect any superior clinical or efficacy outcomes with USAT.[28–30] Published in 2021, the SUNSET SPE study was a randomized trial addressing the question of whether USAT using EKOS catheter is superior to standard multi-side hole CDT catheters for submassive PE patients.[31] Eighty-one patients were randomized in a 1:1 fashion to USAT or SCDT with similar mean lytic dosing protocols between both groups (18 mg over 14 hours). Although significant reductions in the primary outcome, modified Miller score, were observed within each group, there was no statistically significant difference between USAT and SCDT groups (9 $\pm$ 6 vs 10 $\pm$ 6, respectively; P =.76). There was a significant difference in the secondary efficacy endpoint with a mean reduction in RV/LV ratio at 48 hours favoring SCDT group (0.59 $\pm$ 0.42) over the USAT group (– 0.37 $\pm$ 0.34) (P =.01). Major bleeding occurred in two patients in the USAT group (intracranial hemorrhage and vaginal bleeding) and none in the SCDT group.

Novel devices utilizing pharmaco-mechanical CDT (PM-CDT) combine targeted thrombolytic delivery with mechanical thrombectomy to fragment thrombus. Thrombus fragmentation increases the total surface area available for endogenous and exogenous lytic agents to bind fibrin receptors, leading to the enhanced dissolution of the clot.[32] The Bashir Endovascular Catheter (BEC) (Thrombolex Inc, New Britain, PA) represents a new methodology for localized catheter-based delivery of thrombolytics. The 7-French BEC has a spiral-cut infusion basket comprising six mini-infusion catheters with a total of 48 laser-drilled holes that infuse tPA (Fig. 4). The basket comes in long (12.5 cm) and short (10 cm) versions to accommodate PAs of varying lengths.[33] The safety and effectiveness of the PM-CDT Bashir catheter were validated in the recently completed RESCUE trial.

CATHETER-BASED THROMBECTOMY

CBT can be performed to directly decrease the thrombotic burden in pulmonary arteries and thus reduce RV afterload. It is beneficial in patients with contraindications to thrombolysis or those at prohibitive risk for surgical thrombectomy, however, may also be done as an upfront strategy.

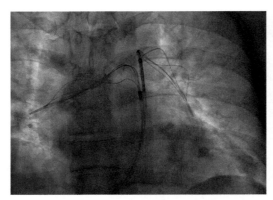

Fig. 4. Fluoroscopic image following placement of two Bashir catheters in right and left pulmonary artery.

There are several devices currently in market, summarized in **Table 2** and further discussed below.

Mechanical Thrombectomy
Inari FlowTriever

The FlowTriever Retrieval/Aspiration System (Inari Medical Inc, Irvine, CA, USA) was FDA-approved for clearance of APE in May 2018. It consists of a large-bore flexible aspiration guide catheter available in 16-, 20-, and 24-Fr sizes. Aspiration is done via a 60-cc custom suction syringe (**Fig. 5**). If there is residual thrombus after initial aspiration attempts, the FlowTriever catheter may then be advanced through the aspiration guide catheter into the thrombus. This catheter consists of three self-expanding nitinol-mesh disks of various sizes that are designed to engage, disrupt, and extract thrombus into the aspiration guide catheter. The device can engage proximal clot well, but due to its large size may not reach distal thrombus. A lot of blood loss may occur during aspiration, however, the FlowSaver system can reduce the blood loss by filtering aspirated thrombi through a 40-micron filtration system and reinfusing blood back into the patient.

To perform thrombectomy with the Inari FlowTriever device, FV access is obtained and pre-close Perclose ProGlide can be placed. Then, after heparin is administered, a catheter such as the Swan-Ganz catheter is advanced to the PA and embedded into the region proximal to the thrombus. This is exchanged for a pigtail catheter and a pulmonary angiogram can then be performed to guide intervention. The catheter is then exchanged for a 24- or 26-Fr large-bore sheath via a stiff 0.035-in guidewire (eg, Amplatz ExtraStiff). The aspiration guide catheter is then advanced over the 0.035-in stiff

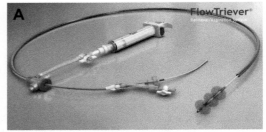

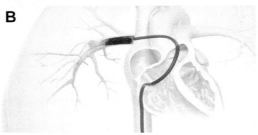

Fig. 5. (A) Inari FlowTriever system consists of a large-bore flexible aspiration guide catheter with a 60-cc custom suction syringe attached to the side tube connector and the FlowTriever catheter with nitinol-mesh disks. (B) The guide catheter is advanced proximal to the occlusive thrombus where aspiration is performed. Permission was obtained by Inari Medical Inc, Irvine, CA.

guidewire just proximal to the occlusive thrombus in the PA (see **Fig. 5**). Aspiration is then performed, after which the device and sheath are removed. The closure is then done via the Perclose if placed; otherwise, a suture may be applied in a figure-of-8 technique till hemostasis is achieved (**Fig. 6**).

The FLARE study was a multicenter single-arm prospective investigational device exemption trial that led to FDA approval of the FlowTriever device. This study evaluated 106 patients aged 18 to 75 with intermediate-risk PE. These patients had symptoms of <14 days duration with proximal PE seen on CT, were hemodynamically stable with heart rate<130 and SBP>90, and RV/LV ratio of >0.9 on CT. The primary efficacy endpoint of RV/LV ratio change from baseline to 48 hours post-procedure showed an average reduction by 0.38 (25.1%) from 1.53 to 1.15.

There was a favorable safety profile with no device-related adverse events, a major bleeding rate of 0.9%, and composite major adverse events of 3.8%.[34]

A single-center retrospective study in 46 patients with either massive or submassive PE showed 100% technical success with a significant reduction in average mean PA pressure (34 – 27 mm Hg) and intraprocedural reduction in oxygen requirements (in 71% of patients). The risk

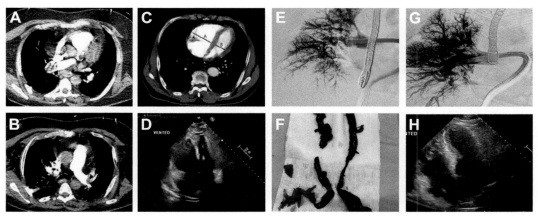

Fig. 6. (Case 2). A 63-year-old male patient developed cardiac arrest on the post-operative day 5 after meningioma resection and was found to have a large burden of proximal emboli in bilateral main pulmonary arteries (A, B). There was an increased right ventricle to left ventricle ratio on computed tomography (C) with severely reduced right ventricle systolic function on echo (D). Due to refractory cardiogenic shock, the patient underwent mechanical thrombectomy with veno-arterial extracorporeal membrane oxygenation support. The initial pulmonary angiogram showed occlusive filling defects in the right interlobar and basilar branches (E). A significant amount of thrombus was removed with the FlowTriever system (F). Perfusion was restored in the right pulmonary artery system (G), and there was an improvement in right ventricle to left ventricle ratio and right ventricle systolic function (H).

of adverse events was <5% with no mortality noted.[35]

A multicenter retrospective analysis of 34 patients with high-risk PE with vasopressor dependence, respiratory failure, or reduced CI had 94% procedural success. There was a significant increase in CI (2.0 –2.4 L/min/m²) and a reduction in mean PA pressure (33 – 25 mm Hg) with no major complications or mortality noted in those with procedural success.[36]

There are multiple upcoming studies that are actively enrolling, including the FLASH registry study, FLAME observational study of patients with massive PE treated with FlowTriever system, and PEERLESS randomized-control trial of FlowTriever versus CDT in patients with intermediate-high-risk PE.

Aspiration Thrombectomy
Penumbra Indigo
The Indigo aspiration system (Penumbra, Inc., Alameda, CA, USA) was FDA-approved for the treatment of PE in December 2019 (Fig. 7). The aspiration thrombectomy catheter is an 8-Fr system (CAT8) and is advanced proximal to the thrombus in the PA via a 0.035-in stiff guidewire. Aspiration is performed and can be repeated multiple times till the thrombus burden has decreased and distal perfusion is restored, making sure to flush between passes. The separator may be used to assist with the clearing of the catheter lumen. There are no means to return aspirated blood and thus there can be

significant blood loss if the catheter is not embedded in the thrombus. More recently, Lightning technology, an intelligent aspiration system that varies the amount of suction based on if the catheter is occlusive in a thrombus or not, has helped optimize clot retrieval while reducing blood loss. There is now also a 12-Fr catheter system (CAT12) that provides a larger lumen for improved aspiration.

To perform thrombectomy with Penumbra Indigo device, femoral or IJ vein access is obtained and pre-close Perclose can be placed. Similar to the steps of Inari FlowTriever, the Swan-Ganz catheter can be advanced to PA, exchanged for a pigtail catheter, and a pulmonary angiogram can be performed. The pigtail catheter is then exchanged for an 8–12-Fr large-bore sheath via a stiff 0.035-in guidewire. Heparin is administered and aspiration is performed, after which the device and sheath are removed. The closure is performed with Perclose or figure-of-8 suture (Fig. 8).

The EXTRACT-PE study was a single-arm investigational drug exemption trial performed on 119 patients with acute submassive PE at 22 sites. Patients had symptoms for <14 days and CT evidence of PE, with SBP > 90, and RV/LV ratio >0.9. Aspiration thrombectomy was performed with a CAT8 device. The primary efficacy endpoint of RV/LV ratio change from baseline to 48 hours post-procedure showed a reduction by 0.43 (27.3%) from 1.47 to 1.04; 39% of patients did not require ICU

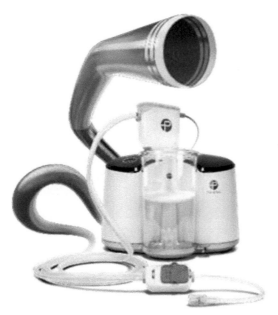

Fig. 7. Penumbra Indigo aspiration system consists of the continuous aspiration thrombectomy (CAT) catheter, Indigo aspiration tubing, and Penumbra engine aspiration source and canister that delivers and maintains vacuum in the catheter. Permission was obtained by Penumbra, Inc., Alameda, CA.

stay, and the median duration of stay in those that stayed in ICU was 1 day.

Major adverse events occurred in 1.7% with 0.8% mortality.[37]

The STRIKE-PE observational study is an ongoing study that will evaluate real-world long-term functional outcomes and safety of the Indigo Aspiration system (12 Fr) in an estimated 600 patients.

AngioVac

The AngioVac (AngioDynamics Inc, Latham, NY, USA) system is a venous drainage system that can be used for retrieval of intravascular materials, including pulmonary emboli, right-heart thrombus/mass, and iliocaval thrombus. This is an extracorporeal circuit with a filter for pump-assisted removal of debris, an 18-Fr inflow cannula (initial iteration had 22-Fr), and a 16–20-Fr outflow cannula that is placed in either IJ or FV. The centrifugal pump generates a flow of up to 4 L/ minute at 2500 to 4000 rpm. There is also the ability to add an oxygenator to the circuit. The inflow cannula is placed just proximal to the intravascular debris or clot and slightly advanced and withdrawn multiple times till debris is removed.

A single-center experience included 12 patients who underwent AngioVac thrombectomy and showed a 58% success rate with 100% success in iliocaval thrombus and only 33% in PE. The effectiveness in PE cases was attributed to the limited steerability of the AngioVac catheter.[38]

Rheolytic Thrombectomy

Rheolytic thrombectomy is performed with the AngioJet device (Boston Scientific, Marlborough, MA, USA). Traditional suction rheolytic

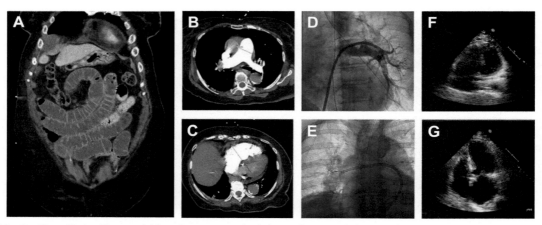

Fig. 8. (Case 3). An 82-year-old female patient with abdominal pain and dyspnea for 2 days was diagnosed with small bowel obstruction requiring urgent surgical intervention (A). Computed tomography angiography chest with large proximal bilateral pulmonary embolism (B) with right ventricle: left ventricle ratio of 1.5 (C). Due to the high risk of general anesthesia in the setting of intermediate-high-risk pulmonary embolism, patient underwent aspiration thrombectomy with Penumbra Indigo device (D, E). Pulmonary artery pressure improved from 42/16 (25) to 31/15 (18) with an improvement in cardiac index from 1.8 to 2.3 L/min/m^2 after thrombectomy. Echo pre-procedure demonstrated increased right ventricle size with reduced function (F) with improvement in right ventricle size and function post-intervention (G). Patient subsequently underwent exploratory laparotomy with resection of small bowel using general anesthesia without complication.

mode consists of retrograde injection of high-pressure ($\sim$10,000 psi) saline jets which then creates a low-pressure zone at the catheter tip via the Bernoulli principle. The saline then recirculates via the Venturi effect and causes thrombus fragmentation. The thrombus can then be aspirated via the catheter. An 8-Fr venous access is needed after which an 8-Fr multipurpose guide catheter is advanced to the PA, and the AngioJet catheter is advanced into the region of thrombus over a 0.035-in guidewire. There is also a power pulse mode where the suction lumen is blocked with a stopcock and a thrombolytic is sprayed into the thrombus.

Rheolytic thrombectomy causes cellular breakdown due to thrombus fragmentation and leads to the release of byproducts such as adenosine and bradykinin into the pulmonary circulation. This has been associated with hypotension, bradycardia, and hypoxia. Thus, there is now a black box warning, and this strategy has fallen out of favor.

Catheter-Based Maceration

Alternatively, the thrombus can be fragmented using a guidewire, balloon, or pigtail catheter that has been advanced to the PA via femoral or IJ venous access. This can rapidly establish partial recanalization of a central embolic occlusion, but has not been well studied and may result in worsening hemodynamics due to distal embolization.[39]

COMPLICATIONS OF ENDOVASCULAR THERAPIES IN PULMONARY EMBOLISM

Given the invasive nature of CDT or percutaneous thrombectomy, there are various associated complications. These can range from access issues such as bleeding and vascular injury to distal thrombus migration, arrhythmias, wire perforation, and PA hemorrhage. Bradycardia and hypotension can occur specifically with rheolytic thrombectomy due to adenosine and bradykinin release from cellular breakdown. However, the morbidity and mortality associated with PE requiring advanced therapies are also high and thus the risks and benefits of such therapies should be weighed.

Consideration should be given to minimize potential complications. Access site complications can be reduced with the utilization of ultrasound-guided, micropuncture access. Additionally, although large-bore access is not required for CDT and closure can safely be performed with manual compression, thrombectomy procedures use much larger catheters (up to 26-Fr with AngioVac). Closure devices such as pre-close (Perclose ProGlide) in combination with manual compression may reduce bleeding complications associated with large-bore venous access.

SUMMARY

In summary, timely risk stratification is critical in managing patients who present with high-risk PE. Incorporating clinical evidence of RV dilatation and dysfunction on imaging, laboratory data, and residual clot burden is key to appropriate risk stratification. In patients presenting with APE who need an escalation of therapy, there have been significant developments in the endovascular devices to manage high-risk patients.

CDT and CBT provide unique and effective strategies for managing patients with high-risk PE with low bleeding and complication rate. Understanding the indications, limitations, and evidence for each approach is critical to success.

CLINICS CARE POINTS

- CDT is safe and effective in the treatment of acute, intermediate-high-risk PE to acutely improve the hemodynamics of right-heart dysfunction compared with systemic anticoagulation.

- Contemporary studies support the use of a lower dose and shorter duration tPA infusion protocol to minimize bleeding risk without compromising efficacy.

- CBT provides an effective non-TPA approach for rapid thrombus approval in the appropriate patient.

DISCLOSURE

Dr A. Darki received research funds from Boston Scientific Corporation.

REFERENCES

1. Giordano NJ, Jansson PS, Young MN, et al. Epidemiology, Pathophysiology, Stratification, and Natural History of Pulmonary Embolism. Tech Vasc Interv Radiol 2017;20(3):135–40.

2. Tritschler T, Kraaijpoel N, Le Gal G, et al. Venous Thromboembolism: Advances in Diagnosis and Treatment. JAMA 2018;320(15):1583–94.

3. Carrier M, Righini M, Wells PS, et al. Subsegmental pulmonary embolism diagnosed by computed tomography: incidence and clinical implications. A

systematic review and meta-analysis of the management outcome studies. J Thromb Haemost 2010;8(8):1716–22.

4. Schulman S, Ageno W, Konstantinides SV. Venous thromboembolism: Past, present and future. Thromb Haemost 2017;117(7):1219–29.

5. Horlander KT, Mannino DM, Leeper KV. Pulmonary embolism mortality in the United States, 1979-1998: an analysis using multiple-cause mortality data. Arch Intern Med 2003;163(14):1711–7.

6. Beckman MG, Hooper WC, Critchley SE, et al. Venous thromboembolism: a public health concern. Am J Prev Med 2010;38(4 Suppl):S495–501.

7. Tagalakis V, Patenaude V, Kahn SR, et al. Incidence of and mortality from venous thromboembolism in a real-world population: the Q-VTE Study Cohort. Am J Med 2013;126(9). 832.e13-e21.

8. Prandoni P, Lensing AWA, Prins MH, et al. Prevalence of Pulmonary Embolism among Patients Hospitalized for Syncope. N Engl J Med 2016;375(16):1524–31.

9. Desai PV, Krepostman N, Collins M, et al. Neurological Complications of Pulmonary Embolism: a Literature Review. Curr Neurol Neurosci Rep 2021;21(10):59.

10. Bauersachs RM. Clinical presentation of deep vein thrombosis and pulmonary embolism. Best Pract Res Clin Haematol 2012;25(3):243–51.

11. Birnbaum A, Esses D, Bijur P, et al. Failure to validate the San Francisco Syncope Rule in an independent emergency department population. Ann Emerg Med 2008;52(2):151–9.

12. Kline JA. Diagnosis and Exclusion of Pulmonary Embolism. Thromb Res 2018;163:207–20.

13. Torbicki A, Perrier A, Konstantinides S, et al. Guidelines on the diagnosis and management of acute pulmonary embolism: the Task Force for the Diagnosis and Management of Acute Pulmonary Embolism of the European Society of Cardiology (ESC). Eur Heart J 2008;29(18):2276–315.

14. Roy PM, Penaloza A, Hugli O, et al. Triaging acute pulmonary embolism for home treatment by Hestia or simplified PESI criteria: the HOME-PE randomized trial. Eur Heart J 2021;42(33):3146–57.

15. Konstantinides SV, Meyer G, Becattini C, et al. 2019 ESC Guidelines for the diagnosis and management of acute pulmonary embolism developed in collaboration with the European Respiratory Society (ERS). Eur Heart J 2020;41(4):543–603.

16. Jaff MR, McMurtry MS, Archer SL, et al. Management of massive and submassive pulmonary embolism, iliofemoral deep vein thrombosis, and chronic thromboembolic pulmonary hypertension: A scientific statement from the american heart association. Circulation 2011. https://doi.org/10.1161/CIR.0b013e318214914f.

17. Jerjes-Sanchez C, Ramírez-Rivera A, de Lourdes García M, et al. Streptokinase and heparin versus heparin alone in massive pulmonary embolism: A randomized controlled trial. J Thromb Thrombolysis 1995. https://doi.org/10.1007/BF01062714.

18. Brailovsky Y, Allen S, Masic D, et al. Risk Stratification of Acute Pulmonary Embolism. Curr Treat Options Cardiovasc Med 2021;23(7):48.

19. Vanni S, Viviani G, Baioni M, et al. Prognostic value of plasma lactate levels among patients with acute pulmonary embolism: the thrombo-embolism lactate outcome study. Ann Emerg Med 2013;61(3):330–8.

20. Frémont B, Pacouret G, Jacobi D, et al. Prognostic value of echocardiographic right/left ventricular end-diastolic diameter ratio in patients with acute pulmonary embolism: results from a monocenter registry of 1,416 patients. Chest 2008;133(2):358–62.

21. Shah BR, Velamakanni SM, Patel A, et al. Analysis of the 60/60 Sign and Other Right Ventricular Parameters by 2D Transthoracic Echocardiography as Adjuncts to Diagnosis of Acute Pulmonary Embolism. Cureus 2021;13(3):e13800.

22. Kucher N, Boekstegers P, Müller OJ, et al. Randomized, controlled trial of ultrasound-assisted catheter-directed thrombolysis for acute intermediate-risk pulmonary embolism. Circulation 2014;129(4):479–86.

23. Piazza G, Hohlfelder B, Jaff MR, et al. A Prospective, Single-Arm, Multicenter Trial of Ultrasound-Facilitated, Catheter-Directed, Low-Dose Fibrinolysis for Acute Massive and Submassive Pulmonary Embolism: The SEATTLE II Study. JACC Cardiovasc Interv 2015;8(10):1382–92.

24. Chiarello MA, Sista AK. Catheter-Directed Thrombolysis for Submassive Pulmonary Embolism. Semin Intervent Radiol 2018;35(2):122–8.

25. Qanadli SD, El Hajjam M, Vieillard-Baron A, et al. New CT index to quantify arterial obstruction in pulmonary embolism: comparison with angiographic index and echocardiography. AJR Am J Roentgenol 2001;176(6):1415–20.

26. Adusumalli S, Geller BJ, Yang L, et al. Trends in catheter-directed thrombolysis and systemic thrombolysis for the treatment of pulmonary embolism. Am Heart J 2019;207:83–5.

27. Tapson VF, Sterling K, Jones N, et al. A Randomized Trial of the Optimum Duration of Acoustic Pulse Thrombolysis Procedure in Acute Intermediate-Risk Pulmonary Embolism: The OPTALYSE PE Trial. JACC Cardiovasc Interv 2018;11(14):1401–10.

28. Liang NL, Avgerinos ED, Marone LK, et al. Comparative Outcomes of Ultrasound-Assisted Thrombolysis and Standard Catheter-Directed Thrombolysis in the Treatment of Acute Pulmonary Embolism. Vasc Endovascular Surg 2016;50(6):405–10.

29. Rao G, Xu H, Wang JJ, et al. Ultrasound-assisted versus conventional catheter-directed thrombolysis

for acute pulmonary embolism: A multicenter comparison of patient-centered outcomes. Vasc Med 2019;24(3):241–7.

30. Kuo WT, Banerjee A, Kim PS, et al. Pulmonary embolism response to fragmentation, embolectomy, and catheter thrombolysis (PERFECT): Initial results from a prospective multicenter registry. Chest 2015. https://doi.org/10.1378/chest.15-0119.

31. Avgerinos ED, Jaber W, Lacomis J, et al. Randomized Trial Comparing Standard Versus Ultrasound-Assisted Thrombolysis for Submassive Pulmonary Embolism: The SUNSET sPE Trial. JACC Cardiovasc Interv 2021;14(12):1364–73.

32. Sista AK, Bhatheja R, Rali P, et al. First-in-Human Study to Assess the Safety and Feasibility of the Bashir Endovascular Catheter for the Treatment of Acute Intermediate-Risk Pulmonary Embolism. Circ Cardiovasc Interv 2021;14(1):e009611.

33. Singh M, Quimby A, Lakhter V, et al. Novel Pharmacomechanical Thrombolysis for Treating Intermediate-Risk Acute Pulmonary Embolism: The Bashir Endovascular Catheter. Tex Heart Inst J 2021;48(5):e217589.

34. Tu T, Toma C, Tapson VF, et al. A Prospective, Single-Arm, Multicenter Trial of Catheter-Directed Mechanical Thrombectomy for Intermediate-Risk Acute Pulmonary Embolism: The FLARE Study. JACC Cardiovasc Interv 2019;12(9):859–69.

35. Wible BC, Buckley JR, Cho KH, et al. Safety and Efficacy of Acute Pulmonary Embolism Treated via Large-Bore Aspiration Mechanical Thrombectomy Using the Inari FlowTriever Device. J Vasc Interv Radiol 2019;30(9):1370–5.

36. Toma C, Khandhar S, Zalewski AM, et al. Percutaneous thrombectomy in patients with massive and very high-risk submassive acute pulmonary embolism. Catheter Cardiovasc Interv 2020;96(7):1465–70.

37. Sista AK, Horowitz JM, Tapson VF, et al. Indigo Aspiration System for Treatment of Pulmonary Embolism: Results of the EXTRACT-PE Trial. JACC Cardiovasc Interv 2021;14(3):319–29.

38. D'Ayala M, Worku B, Gulkarov I, et al. Factors Associated with Successful Thrombus Extraction with the AngioVac Device: An Institutional Experience. Ann Vasc Surg 2017;38:242–7.

39. Schmitz-Rode T, Janssens U, Duda SH, et al. Massive pulmonary embolism: percutaneous emergency treatment by pigtail rotation catheter. J Am Coll Cardiol 2000;36(2):375–80.

Mechanical Circulatory Support and Critical Care Management of High-Risk Acute Pulmonary Embolism

Aaron A. Sifuentes, MD[a], Ghazaleh Goldar, MD[b],
Ahmad A. Abdul-Aziz, MD[c], Ran Lee, MD[b],
Supriya Shore, MD, MSCS[a],*

KEYWORDS

• Pulmonary embolism • Right ventricular failure • Mechanical circulatory support

KEY POINTS

- Acute pulmonary embolism has a high mortality rate driven by acute right ventricular failure that remains clinically challenging to assess and manage.
- Critical care management of high-risk acute pulmonary embolism includes early detection, optimization of volume status, afterload management with vasopressors, inotropic support, and early anticoagulation therapy with thrombolytic therapy.
- Mechanical circulatory support, including percutaneous and surgical approaches, is emerging as treatment options for refractory shock due to acute right ventricular failure in the setting of high-risk acute pulmonary embolism, but additional studies are needed.

INTRODUCTION

Hemodynamically significant pulmonary embolism (PE) remains a widely prevalent, underdiagnosed condition associated with mortality rates as high as 30%.[1] The main driver of poor outcomes is acute right ventricular failure (RVF) that remains clinically challenging to diagnose and manage. Treatment of high-risk (or massive) acute PE has traditionally included systemic anticoagulation and thrombolysis. Over the past few years, a renewed interest in mechanical circulatory support (MCS; both percutaneous and surgical) for acute RVF has emerged, increasing viable treatment options for high-risk acute PE. In this narrative review, the authors discuss the pathophysiology of acute RVF, clinical features, and management of ensuing shock including MCS in patients with high-risk acute PE.

PATHOPHYSIOLOGY OF RIGHT VENTRICULAR FAILURE IN ACUTE PULMONARY EMBOLISM

Normal Right Ventricular Anatomy and Physiology

The right ventricle (RV) is a thin, compliant wall with a predominantly longitudinal myofibril arrangement as compared with a thicker walled left ventricle (LV) with circumferential myofibrils. RV function is governed by preload (systemic venous return), afterload (pulmonary artery [PA] pressure), myocardial contractility of the RV free wall and interventricular septum, and pericardial compliance. The RV functions as a low-pressure, high-volume system as it couples with the low-pressure, high-compliance pulmonary circuit.[2–4] Accordingly, the RV uses one-sixth the amount of energy used by the LV, and

[a] University of Michigan Department of Internal Medicine, 1500 East Medical Center Drive, 3116 Taubman Center, SPC 5368, Ann Arbor, MI 48109-5368, USA; [b] Cleveland Clinic Department of Cardiovascular Medicine, Heart, Vascular, and Thoracic Institute, 9500 Euclid Avenue, Mail Code J3-4, Cleveland, OH 44195, USA; [c] Inova Heart and Vascular Institute, 3300 Gallows Road, Critical Care Medicine, Falls Church, VA 22042, USA
* Corresponding author. University of Michigan, NCRC 16-169C, 2800 Plymouth Road, SPC 2800, Ann Arbor, MI 48109-2800.
E-mail address: shores@med.umich.edu

Intervent Cardiol Clin 12 (2023) 323–338
https://doi.org/10.1016/j.iccl.2023.03.004
2211-7458/23/© 2023 Elsevier Inc. All rights reserved.

normal RV function is primarily driven by afterload.[3]

Pathophysiology of Right Ventricular Failure in the Setting of Acute Pulmonary Embolism

In acute PE, there is a rapid increase in pulmonary vascular resistance (PVR) that results in a sudden increase in RV afterload. The mechanism for increased PVR in acute PE is multifactorial, including direct blood flow impedance, local hypoxia-induced vasoconstriction, and platelet/thrombin-induced release of vasoactive peptides.[5] The cascade of events that then leads to RVF includes decreased RV stoke volume, increased RV wall tension, and RV dilation[3] (Fig. 1).

Right ventricle stroke volume

Owing to its anatomy, the RV is particularly sensitive to sudden changes in afterload. A small increase in RV afterload can cause a disproportionate and exponentially large decrease in RV stroke volume. A reduction in RV stroke volume leads to decreased RV cardiac output (CO), RV dilation, and decreased LV preload, all subsequently leading to a decrease in LV CO.[3]

Increased right ventricle wall tension

The sharp rise in pressure from increased RV afterload in acute PE results in increased RV wall tension. With increased wall tension comes an increased oxygen demand necessitating increased coronary blood flow. However, unlike the LV, coronary perfusion of the RV occurs both during systole and diastole.[3] The pressure-overloaded RV increases RV end-diastolic pressure, which hinders coronary perfusion pressures and coronary blood flow, placing the RV at high risk for ischemia.[2,3]

Right ventricle dilation

RV dilation in the setting of acute PE occurs both as a direct effect of increased RV afterload and as an indirect effect from decreased RV CO causing venous congestion. This RV volume and pressure overload increases transmural pressure across the interventricular septum causing a leftward shift of the interventricular septal shift due to pericardial constraint. Septal deviation then increases LV end-diastolic pressure and decreases LV preload, ultimately causing a decrease in LV function and CO.[2,3,6]

DIAGNOSIS OF ACUTE RIGHT VENTRICULAR FAILURE AND SHOCK

The initial assessment is based on patient symptoms and hemodynamic status as assessed on physical examination (Table 1). Further risk stratification can be performed by laboratory testing looking specifically for acute renal and liver injury from an elevated jugular venous pressure (JVP) due to RV dysfunction. In addition, elevated natriuretic peptides (B-type natriuretic peptide [BNP]/N-terminal prohormone of B-type natriuretic peptide [NT-proBNP]) and troponin levels both correlate with RV dysfunction and may portend a poor

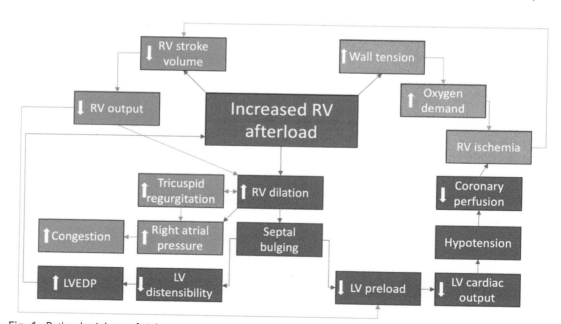

Fig. 1. Pathophysiology of right ventricular failure in the setting of increased right ventricular afterload. LV, left ventricle; LVEDP, LV end-diastolic pressure; RV, right ventricle.

Table 1
Typical symptoms and physical exam findings in acute pulmonary embolism

Typical Symptoms of PE	Physical Examination Findings in PE Raising Concern for RVF
• Dyspnea • Chest pain • Palpitations • Dizziness • Syncope • Tachypnea	• Elevated JVP • Parasternal heave • Holosystolic tricuspid regurgitation murmur • Right sided 3rd heart sound • Evidence of hypoperfusion: hypotension, tachycardia, diaphoresis, cool extremities

MANAGEMENT OF ACUTE INTERMEDIATE AND HIGH-RISK PULMONARY EMBOLISM

Approximately 8% of patients with PE present in shock (ie, high-risk PE) with a mortality rate of 30% to 50% in the first week,[14] and patients who present with intermediate-risk PE have a mortality rate of up to 25% in the same time span.[15] Accordingly, management of intermediate-risk and high-risk PE requires timely, attentive, and intensive critical care due to the hemodynamic collapse that can follow. Management of these patients typically involves concomitant diagnostic testing using bedside echo or CT, anticoagulation, and resuscitation. In severe cases of RVF, percutaneous and surgical options can be considered in addition to medical treatment to help improve outcomes.

prognosis.[7–9] Electrocardiogram (ECG) findings of right heart strain are nonspecific and have limited sensitivity, though can include an S1Q3T3 pattern that suggests right heart strain in an acute PE (Fig. 2).[10] Finally, imaging data based on computed tomography (CT) and/or echocardiogram are used to confirm a diagnosis of PE and assess for RVF. A meta-analysis of CT findings in acute PE found that a ratio of the RV to LV (RV/LV) ≥ 1 in patients with PE was associated with an approximately 2.5-fold increase in all-cause mortality.[11] Based on these parameters, PE can broadly be classified as low-risk, intermediate-risk (submassive), or high-risk (massive). Intermediate-risk PE has evidence of right heart strain on imaging (CT [Fig. 3] or echocardiography) and biomarker studies (troponin and BNP/NT-proBNP levels). Echocardiographic findings of right heart strain are detailed in Fig. 4.[12] High-risk PE denotes the presence of hemodynamic instability, that is, persistent hypotension with systolic blood pressure less than 90 or hemodynamics requiring vasopressor support.[13]

MEDICAL MANAGEMENT OF ACUTE PULMONARY EMBOLISM
Preload Management
Acute RVF in the setting of PE leads to a low CO state and cardiogenic shock. Careful assessment of RV preload by clinically assessing JVP is paramount. The placement of a PA catheter in patients with PE only for monitoring central venous pressure (CVP) is not recommended due to risk for clot dislodgement and higher procedure-associated risks. In addition, contemporary data suggest that CVP does not reliably reflect fluid responsiveness in patients with an acute illness.[16]

The basic tenet of fluid resuscitation in all patients with acute RVF has been challenged by several studies[17–19] as excessive volume loading can lead to overdistention of the RV and worsening of the CO due to mechanisms highlighted previously.[20] Accordingly, targeting a CVP of 8 to 12 mm Hg is recommended. Volume loading with a modest (≤500 mL) amount of fluid can be considered when the CVP is lower to help

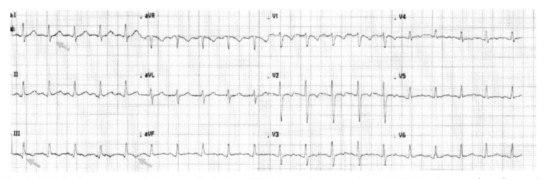

Fig. 2. EKG findings in Acute Pulmonary Embolism. EKG above demonstrates a S1Q3T3 pattern, with an S wave in lead I (*arrow* in lead I), Q wave in lead III (*left arrow* in lead III), and inverted T wave in lead III (*right arrow* in lead III). (Image from "Pulmonary Embolism – EKG findings".[10])

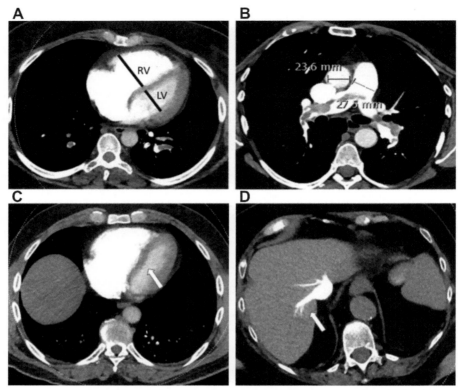

Fig. 3. CT findings of right heart strain. (A) Increased RV to LV ratio and measurements, (B) Increased main PA measurements compared to the aorta, (C) bowing of interventricular septum into the LV (indicated by *arrow*), (D) contrast reflux into IVC (indicated by *arrow*). (Image from "Right heart strain assessment on CTPA following acute pulmonary embolism."[70])

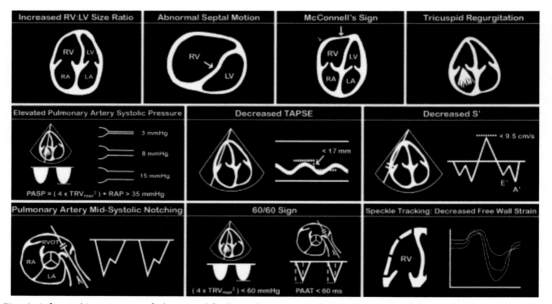

Fig. 4. Infographic summary of ultrasound findings that suggest right heart strain. McConnell's sign refers to RV mid-wall akinesia with apical sparing. (Reproduced from Alerhand S, Sundaram T, Gottlieb M. What are the echocardiographic findings of acute right ventricular strain that suggest pulmonary embolism?.Anaesthesia Critical Care & Pain Medicine. 2021;40(2):100852. Copyright © 2021 Elsevier Masson SAS. All rights reserved.)

increase the CO.[21] For patients with a higher CVP, decongestion should be strongly considered in an attempt to restore RV geometry and improve LV filling. In a recent randomized trial, normotensive patients with intermediate-risk PE randomized to furosemide were more likely to have normalized hemodynamic and respiratory status at 24 hours compared with placebo.[19] In hypotensive patients with high-risk PE who are clearly volume overloaded, diuretics should not be withheld but measures to support blood pressure with vasopressors should be concomitantly provided, as reducing central venous congestion will help reduce RV dilation and improve CO.

Respiratory Support

Supplemental oxygen should be promptly provided for patients with oxygen saturation less than 90%. Intubation and mechanical ventilation should be reserved only for acute PE patients with severe refractory hypoxemia and hemodynamic instability as induction with sedation and muscle relaxation before intubation can cause peripheral vasoplegia, worsening RV preload and RV perfusion. In one case series, hemodynamic collapse occurred in 19% of patients during general anesthesia induction for pulmonary embolectomy.[22] Therefore, when indicated, intubation should be performed with close hemodynamic monitoring. Empiric initiation of vasopressors should be considered before administration of induction agents to ameliorate the adverse hemodynamic consequences of induction and the effects of positive pressure ventilation on an injured RV. Ideal agents for induction in patients with PE include etomidate or ketamine as they do not influence hemodynamics substantially, and agents such as propofol should be avoided given their vasodilatory effect.[23] Alternatively, strategies such as awake fiberoptic intubation may be used when feasible.[24] Ultimately, if the patient is a candidate for thrombolysis, the best approach may be to delay intubation while pursuing immediate thrombolysis.

Apart from risks associated with induction, episodes of apnea and hypoxemia after induction can cause an increase in PVR. Therefore, apneic time should be minimized, and a skilled provider should intubate using technology such as video laryngoscopy when available. Large tidal volumes lead to an increase in intrathoracic pressure causing a drop in RV preload and increase PVR.[25] Thus, aggressive bag-mask ventilation should be avoided and tidal volumes of 6 to 8 mL/kg ideal body weight should be used.[20,26]

Following intubation, mechanical ventilation settings must be closely monitored and adjusted to minimize unfavorable hemodynamic effects. Targeted ventilation strategies in patients with acute RVF (as seen in patients with high-risk PE) aim to avoid increasing PVR. These strategies include the use of low tidal volumes, minimizing positive end expiratory pressure, and preventing hypoxemia and acidemia.[27,28]

Afterload Management

For patients who remain hypotensive despite initial fluid resuscitation or are hypotensive and volume overloaded, vasopressors and inotropic agents are indicated (Table 2). Vasopressors help support blood pressure, improve perfusion to organs, and improve coronary blood flow to the pressure overloaded RV. Commonly used vasopressors for RVF and shock include norepinephrine and epinephrine. The use of norepinephrine in cardiogenic shock secondary to acute PE improves ventricular systolic interaction and coronary perfusion, without increasing PVR.[29] Norepinephrine acts predominantly via α1-receptor stimulation causing systemic vasoconstriction, with mild β1-receptor stimulation causing a small increase in inotropy. Studies with epinephrine are limited in isolated RVF. Epinephrine also acts via α1 receptors, though has more β1-receptor activity leading to increased inotropy. Overall, epinephrine also seems to have minimal effect on PVR.[20] For patients' refractory to high-dose norepinephrine or epinephrine, vasopressin can be added for hemodynamic support. Vasopressin increases systemic vascular resistance (SVR) with no change in PVR due to the lack of vasopressin receptors within pulmonary vasculature.[30] Phenylephrine use is not recommended due to the theoretical risk of increasing PVR[31]; however, studies of this drug in acute PE are lacking.

Contractile support

For patients with adequate preload and vasopressor support who continue to show signs of low CO, inotropes are indicated. Markers of low CO include decreased urine output, altered mental status, cool extremities, poor capillary refill, and elevated lactic acid levels. When inotropes are indicated, dobutamine is the agent of choice. As dobutamine causes some peripheral vasodilation, it should be used with vasopressors if systemic hypoperfusion is present. Milrinone is not recommended in acute RVF and shock secondary to PE because of concomitant vasodilation it causes with a substantially longer half-life compared with dobutamine.

Table 2
Medical treatment strategies in high-risk acute pulmonary embolism

	Strategy	Indications	Adverse Effects
Preload optimization	Target CVP of 8–12.	In patients with low–normal CVP IV fluid resuscitation with saline or Ringer's lactate (500 mL over 15–30 min) is recommended. In patients with high CVP diuretics are recommended	Excessive fluid resuscitation will lead to overdistention of the RV and worsening ventricular interdependence. Excessive diuresis will cause underfilling of the RV and reduce cardiac output
Norepinephrine	Vasopressor of choice in PE. Increases SVR without increasing the PVR. Limited increase in RV inotropy. Improved coronary perfusion gradient	Hemodynamic instability associated with hypotension, RVF, and signs of end organ dysfunction	Excessive vasoconstriction can worsen tissue ischemia
Epinephrine	Increases SVR with minimal effect on PVR. Increase in RV inotropy	Hemodynamic instability associated with hypotension, RVF, and signs of end organ dysfunction	Excessive vasoconstriction can worsen tissue ischemia. Increased risk for developing arrhymias
Vasopressin	Increases SVR without increasing PVR. No effect on RV inotropy	Patients' refractory to high-dose norepinephrine or epinephrine	Usually well tolerated
Phenylephrine	Increases SVR, but can also increase PVR	—	Can increase PVR and NOT recommended
Dobutamine	Inotrope of choice in RVF. Lowers filling pressures	Normotensive, preload optimized patients with low cardiac index	Can exacerbate V/Q mismatch by redistributing the flow from partially obstructed pulmonary vessels to unobstructed ones
Anticoagulation	Inhibits platelet aggregation facilitating clot dissolution. UFH, LMWH, and NOACs are viable choices	Initiated promptly in patients with a high or intermediate clinical probability of PE while awaiting confirmatory testing result. UFH is preferred in patients with hemodynamic instability	Major bleeding. Heparin-induced thrombocytopenia. Dose adjustments needed for LMWH and NOAC in patients with poor renal function

Systemic thrombolysis	Activates proteases that cleave plasminogen into plasmin, leading to clot dissolution. Can be administered systemically via peripheral IV or directed locally via catheter	Used in patients with high-risk or intermediate-risk PE, who have hemodynamic instability or have failed medical therapy. Benefit is greatest when given within 48 hours of presentation	Major bleeding
Oxygen supplementation	Adequate oxygenation can help minimize hypoxemia or apnea induced increases in PVR	Provided for patients with oxygen saturation <90%	Intubation and mechanical ventilation can decrease RV preload and increase PVR. Aggressive bag-mask ventilation should be avoided, as large tidal volumes decrease RV preload
Pulmonary vasodilators	Inhaled pulmonary vasodilators help lower PVR and optimize V/Q mismatch, with minimal effect on SVR	Parenteral pulmonary vasodilators are not recommended. Inhaled vasodilators can be used in hemodynamically unstable patients	Parenteral pulmonary vasodilators can cause systemic hypotension and hypoperfusion. Limited studies on use of inhaled pulmonary vasodilators

Abbreviations: CVP, central venous pressure; LMWH, low molecular weight heparin; NOACs, non-vitamin K oral anticoagulants; PE, pulmonary embolism; PVR, pulmonary vascular resistance; UFH, unfractionated heparin; V/Q, ventilation perfusion ratio.

However, data on inotropic support for RVF with dobutamine and milrinone in the setting of an acute PE are limited to animal models.[32]

Anticoagulation

According to the 2019 European Society of Cardiology (ESC) guidelines, anticoagulation with either unfractionated heparin (UFH) or low molecular weight heparin (LMWH) should be initiated promptly in patients with a high or intermediate clinical probability of PE while awaiting confirmatory testing results.[33] Benefits of heparin extend to reducing PVR by inhibiting platelet aggregation facilitating clot dissolution and inhibiting the release of vasoactive substances.[34,35] Currently, LMWH is preferred over UFH due to the lower risk profile of inducing major bleeding or heparin-induced thrombocytopenia.[33] However, UFH continues to be the first-line agent in patients with overt hemodynamic instability or high risk of hemodynamic compromise who might be candidates for reperfusion treatments.[33] Caution should be made while using LMWH in obese patients (dose adjustment needed) and in patients with creatinine clearance ≤ 30 mL/min. When oral anticoagulation is started, guidelines recommend the use of a non-vitamin K oral anticoagulant (NOAC) over vitamin K antagonists.[33] The early administration of such agents has been shown to reduce mortality in patients with acute PE.[36] In addition, therapeutic anticoagulation has been shown to reduce the rate of recurrent venous thromboembolism, which is another significant factor in the mortality of patients with PE.[37,38] Observational studies have shown a reduction of RV/LV ratio in patients with acute PE who are treated only with anticoagulation.[39] However, composite data from several trials have failed to show a correlation between reduction in RV/LV ratio and prevention of clinical decompensation.[39] These findings have sparked interest in exploring advanced therapeutic and mechanical strategies in combination with anticoagulation.

Systemic Thrombolysis

Thrombolytic treatment helps dissolve blood clots by activation of serine proteases which ultimately leads to cleavage of plasminogen into plasmin. These agents are administered either systemically via peripheral intravenous (IV) or directed with an invasive catheter at the site of the blood clot.[40] For hemodynamically unstable patients with high-risk PE, systemic thrombolysis can be performed faster than catheter-directed thrombolysis. For such patients, once a diagnosis of PE is confirmed, systemic thrombolysis should be initiated in the absence of absolute contraindications[15] (Table 3). For hemodynamically unstable patients with contraindications to systemic thrombolysis or those who fail to improve with thrombolysis, embolectomy (catheter directed or surgical) is the next step.

In studies of patients with intermediate-risk PE, systemic thrombolytic therapy when compared with UFH alone improved pulmonary obstruction, pulmonary arterial pressure (PAP), and PVR at a faster rate. This improvement reduces the RV strain and leads to a reduction in RV dilation that can be observed in an echocardiogram.[41] Although benefits are the most when given within 48 hours of presentation, patients can still benefit for up to 14 days from presentation.[42] The efficacy of systemic thrombolysis in patients with intermediate-risk PE was investigated in the Pulmonary Embolism Thrombolysis trial, which showed that normotensive patients with intermediate-risk PE who received a single IV bolus of tenecteplase had a reduced risk for hemodynamic compromise. However, the risk of bleeding was higher as compared with placebo with no difference in mortality.[41] Nevertheless, mortality benefit with thrombolysis in PE patients with RVF has been demonstrated in two meta-analyses.[43,44] Owing to an increased risk of major bleeding, contraindications should be thoroughly reviewed before administration.[43] More recently, there has been an emerging interest in half-dose thrombolysis. In the MOPETT trial, low-dose tissue plasminogen activator (tPA) (0.5 mg/kg – max 50 mg alteplase) plus anticoagulation reduced the incidence of pulmonary hypertension and of the composite outcome of pulmonary hypertension or recurrent PE compared with anticoagulation alone.[45] Currently, data are limited regarding the long-term benefits of using systemic thrombolytics, and the ESC 2019 guidelines do not support routine utilization of thrombolytics in all PE patients.[33]

Pulmonary Vasodilators

Pulmonary vasoconstriction contributes significantly to the development of RVF in patients with acute PE. This vasoconstriction is the result of mechanical obstruction of the pulmonary vessels as well as other factors such as endothelial effects, tissue hypoxia, and humoral factors released as a result of platelet activation.[46] Vigorous clinical studies evaluating the use of pulmonary vasodilators in acute PE patients to decrease the PAP and PVR are lacking, and the evidence is limited

Table 3
Absolute and relative contraindications to systemic thrombolysis Relative Contraindications Absolute Contraindication

Relative Contraindications	Absolute Contraindications
• Age >75 years old • Current use of anticoagulation • Pregnancy • Noncompressible vascular punctures • Traumatic or prolonged cardiopulmonary resuscitation (>10 min) • Recent (within 2–4 wk) internal bleeding • Chronic, severe, poorly controlled hypertension (systolic blood pressure [SBP] >180 mm Hg or diastolic blood pressure [DBP] >110 mm Hg) • Dementia • Remote (>3 months) ischemic stroke • Major surgery within 3 wk	• Prior intracranial hemorrhage • Known intracranial arteriovenous malformation • Known malignant intracranial neoplasm • Ischemic stroke within 3 mo • Suspected aortic dissection • Active bleeding • Recent surgery (within 3 mo) of the spinal canal or brain • Recent closed-head or facial trauma with evidence of bony fracture or brain injury

to case series or animal models.[46] Parenteral pulmonary vasodilators carry the risk of systemic hypotension and hypoperfusion and can contribute to the worsening of ventilation/perfusion (V/Q) mismatch in the pulmonary system and are therefore avoided.[46] The guidelines thus do not support the use of pulmonary vasodilators in the setting of acute PE.[33] However, for hemodynamically unstable patients, inhaled pulmonary vasodilators (ie,. inhaled nitric oxide and epoprostenol) may be used. Inhaled vasodilators cause minimal systemic hypotension, lower PVR, and optimize V/Q mismatch. There are limited studies supporting the use of inhaled nitric oxide in acute PE to improve hemodynamics,[47] and there is no evidence supporting the efficacy or safety of such agents.

Interventional (percutaneous) mechanical circulatory support for acute right ventricular failure in the setting of acute pulmonary embolism
In the contemporary era, several percutaneous devices have emerged, which provide temporary MCS to the RV. These include Impella RP, Tandem-Heart right ventricular assist device (TH-RVAD) or Protek, and veno-arterial extracorporeal membrane oxygenation (VA-ECMO). Table 4 summarizes the percutaneous RV MCS systems used in RVF. MCS in patients with acute PE is indicated for patients with refractory shock (ie, not responding to thrombolysis/anticoagulation in patients with preload/afterload optimization and inotropic support). Challenges to using these devices in patients with acute PE include clot dislodgement, vascular complications, infections, device migration, and fracture of individual elements.[48–50]

Veno-Arterial Extracorporeal Membrane Oxygenation
The ESC 2019 guidelines endorse ECMO for patients with high-risk PE and refractory circulatory collapse or cardiac arrest. As collapse in high-risk PE patients is due to circulatory failure and not respiratory failure, VA-ECMO is preferred over venovenous-ECMO. VA-ECMO reduces RV preload and improves systemic oxygenation by displacing venous blood from the right atrium (RA) into an oxygenator and back into the arterial circulation via the femoral artery (Fig. 5). As it displaces blood from the venous system into the arterial system, VA-ECMO increases LV afterload which can have clinical implications in patients with reduced LV function. This is usually not of concern for patients with acute RVF due to high-risk PE.

VA-ECMO is deployed percutaneously via an extracorporeal centrifugal pump. The arterial access sheath size ranges from 15F to 21F and the venous access sheath size ranges from 21F to 25F.[51] Alternatively, veno-veno-arterial ECMO (VV-A-ECMO) can be used to drain blood from both the RA and PA. By doing so, VV-A-ECMO reduces RV afterload and allows time for recovery of the failed ventricle. Complications of ECMO include limb ischemia, stroke, and intracranial hemorrhage.[52]

There are limited, low-quality clinical data on the efficacy and hemodynamic changes associated with VA-ECMO in the setting of acute RVF due to high-risk PE. In one of the largest single-center studies, early use of VA-ECMO in 21 high-risk PE patients with end-organ dysfunction was associated with a 95% survival rate at 90 days.[53] In a recent meta-analysis, VA-ECMO

Table 4
Acute percutaneous right ventricular mechanical circulatory support systems for isolated right ventricular failure

Device	Inlet	Outlet	Sheath Size	Flow Range (L/Min)	Effect on RA	Effect on Mean PA	Effect on PCWP	Effect on CO	Effect on MAP	Advantages	Disadvantages
Impella RP	Right atrium	Pulmonary artery	23F	2–4	↓	↑	↑	↑	No change	Easy deployment Directly bypasses the RV	Inability to oxygenate the blood Bleeding Hemolysis
TH-RVAD or Protek Duo	Right atrium	Pulmonary artery	29F or 31F sheath	2–4	↓	↑	↑	↑	No change	Oxygenates blood Directly bypasses the RV	Large sheath size
VA-ECMO	Right atrium	Femoral artery	Arterial: 15F–21F Venous: 21F–25F	2–6	↓	No change	↓	No change	↑↑	Oxygenates blood	Bleeding

Abbreviations: CO, cardiac output; MAP, mean arterial pressure; PA, pulmonary artery; PCWP, pulmonary capillary wedge pressure; RA, right atrium.

Extracorporeal Oxygenation Membrane (ECMO)

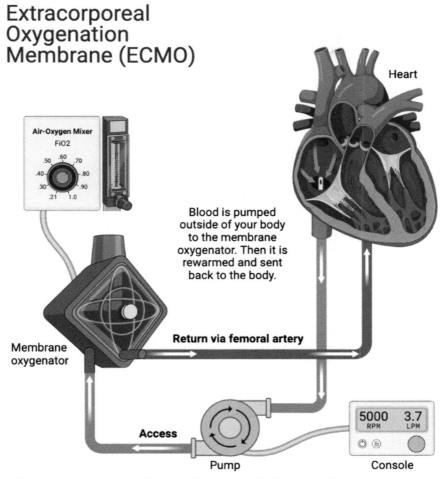

Air-Oxygen Mixer
FiO2

Blood is pumped outside of your body to the membrane oxygenator. Then it is rewarmed and sent back to the body.

Heart

Return via femoral artery

Membrane oxygenator

Access

Pump

5000 RPM   3.7 LPM

Console

Fig. 5. VA-ECMO displacing venous blood from the RA, oxygenating it via a membrane oxygenator, and returning it to the arterial circulation via the femoral artery. (Template adapted from Dr. Yevgeniy Brailovsky from Sidney Kimmel School of Medicine.)

use in patients with high-risk PE did not correlate with improved short-term survival. There was low-quality evidence to suggest VA-ECMO may be beneficial in patients ≤ 60 years or in those who have undergone surgical embolectomy.[54]

Impella RP

The Impella RP (Abiomed Inc, Danvers, MA) is a micro-axial flow catheter that can be used to directly bypass the RV in the setting of acute RVF by diverting blood from the RA to the PA. It uses a 22F impeller mounted on an 11F catheter (**Fig. 6**).[6] To deliver this device, a single venous access site is established with the right femoral vein being the most common site. The device is then introduced into the PA using a 23F venous peel-away sheath with a 0.018″ wire that is used as a monorail system. Once correct positioning is confirmed, the 23F sheath is

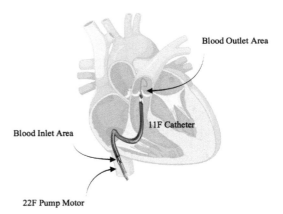

Blood Outlet Area

Blood Inlet Area

11F Catheter

22F Pump Motor

Fig. 6. Impella RP Device. Inlet area from the RA with outlet area in the PA, delivering blood from the RA to the PA using an axial flow pump motor. (Created with BioRender.com.)

replaced with a staged 11F to 23F repositioning sheath.[6] The safety and efficacy of Impella RP has largely been investigated in the context of refractory RVF due to acute myocardial infarction or post-cardiotomy syndrome.[55,56] This includes the RECOVER RIGHT trial that showed immediate improvement in hemodynamics with a reduction in CVP, increase in CO, and ability to wean inotropes and vasopressors. Evidence examining the use of Impella RP for acute RVF in high-risk PE is limited to the case reports that suggest it may be a viable option in patients with refractory shock.[57] Infrequently, worsening tricuspid or pulmonary valve dysfunction may occur.[55] Of note, Impella RP cannot oxygenate blood.

TandemHeart RIGHT VENTRICULAR ASSIST DEVICE AND PROTEK DUO

TH-RVAD is an extracorporeal centrifugal flow pump that also directly bypasses the RV by displacing blood from the RA to PA. To implant the device, two 21F venous access sites are needed for the RA (inflow cannula) and PA (outflow cannula), usually via the left and right femoral veins, respectively. Blood drained from the RA is delivered to a centrifugal pump, where it gets oxygenated and returned to the PA.[6] Femoral venous access can be challenging in patients with existing thrombosis, infection, or inferior vena cava filters.[58] The placement of the outflow cannula can be challenging in patients with large torsos (>58 cm distance between femoral vein and fifth intercostal space), and in these cases, the right internal jugular vein (IJ) may be used.[6] The use of the IJ as an access site led to the development of the Protek Duo dual-lumen cannula. This cannula includes two lumens within a single 29 or 31F cannula. This allows for the placement of the inflow outlet with a series of vents within the RA and superior vena cava and the outflow outlet with a fenestrated distal tip within the main PA (Fig. 7). A key difference between the Impella-RP and TH-RVAD is that the TH-RVAD can be used to oxygenate blood by splicing an oxygenator into the circuit and converting it into an oxyRVAD.

Efficacy of the TH-RVAD was retrospectively studied in 46 patients with RVF. The results showed improved hemodynamics, as there was an increase in MAP, CO, oxygen saturation, and a decrease in RA and PA systolic pressures.[6] Another study highlighted a higher mortality rate among patients with delayed TH-RVAD placement, promoting earlier utilization of such devices.[59] Data on the use of these devices in patients with high-risk PE are limited to small case series.[60]

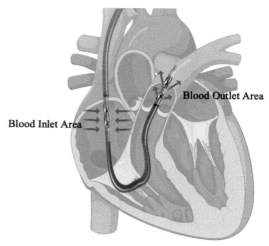

Fig. 7. Protek Duo dual-lumen cannula. Inflow outlet with a series of vents within the RA and superior vena cava and the outflow outlet with a fenestrated distal tip in the main PA. (Created with BioRender.com.)

SURGICAL MECHANICAL CIRCULATORY SUPPORT FOR ACUTE RIGHT VENTRICULAR FAILURE IN THE SETTING OF ACUTE PULMONARY EMBOLISM
Surgically Implanted Right Ventricular Assist Device

Surgical RVADs are rarely used for acute RVF in patients with high-risk PE and are limited for patients who have failed medical management and typical percutaneous support devices are contraindicated. Surgical RVADs include extracorporeal centrifugal pumps (CentriMag, St. Jude, Minneapolis, MN) or durable LVADs placed in the RV position. These devices are implanted via thoracotomy or open sternotomy to allow for direct cannulation of the RA and PA, which allows bypass of the failing RV[61] (Fig. 8). The benefit of surgical implantation is the ability to use short, large-bore cannulas (rather than long small bore cannulas used in peripheral RVADs) that allow for higher flows and improved RV decompression.[62] The major disadvantage for a surgical approach is the need for an invasive procedure and difficulty with identifying appropriate timing of surgical intervention.[63] RVADs unload the failing RV, allowing for improved flow into the PA as well as decreasing RV wall tension to decrease RV myocardial oxygen demand and improve myocyte recovery.[64] However, it is theorized that RVADs may increase PVR due to improved blood flow to the PA, although studies are limited.[65] Although emerging as an option for the management of RVF, there are limited data on efficacy of RVAD use in RVF related to acute PE. Existing studies are based on RVF due to LV

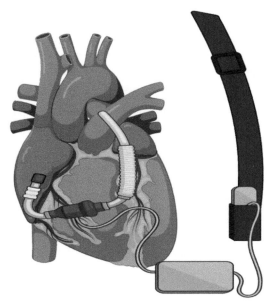

Fig. 8. Surgically implanted right ventricular assist device (RVAD) with inlet into the right atrium and outlet into the main pulmonary artery. (Created with Bio-Render.com.)

dysfunction, chronic pulmonary hypertension, myocardial infraction, or post-cardiotomy.[66] There are limited case reports of surgical RVADs used specifically in the setting of acute PE with promising results, though further studies are needed.[67] The strongest data supporting RVAD use in acute RVF are with the CentriMag (continuous centrifugal rotary flow device), which can be used as an isolated RVAD for up to 30 days, allowing up to 6 to 10 L/min blood flow.[61,62,66] Further studies are needed to evaluate the use of durable RVADs for long-term support.

Pulmonary Embolism Response Team
Given the high mortality rate and importance of expeditious management of high-risk and intermediate-risk acute PE, several institutions have implemented PE response teams (PERTs). PERTs are composed of multidisciplinary team members across several specialties, including cardiology, intensive care, interventional radiology, vascular medicine, hematology, and cardiothoracic surgery, allowing for timely discussion and potential intervention with advanced therapies.[68] Registry data and single-center studies with PERT implementation have shown an increase in the use of advanced therapies for management of high-risk acute PE, decreased complications, and overall improved mortality.[68,69]

CLINICS CARE POINTS

- Diuretics help restore RV geometry and improve LV filling, resulting in improved hemodynamics in patients with high-risk acute PE. In hypotensive patients with high-risk PE who are volume overloaded, diuretics should not be withheld but measures to support blood pressure with vasopressors should be concomitantly provided, as reducing central venous congestion will help reduce RV dilation and improve cardiac output.

- In patients with high-risk acute PE who are mechanically ventilated, ventilation strategies are aimed to avoid increasing pulmonary vascular resistance that can worsen RV failure. These strategies include the use of low tidal volumes, minimizing positive end expiratory pressure, and preventing hypoxemia and acidemia.

- Current guidelines do not support the use of pulmonary vasodilators in the setting of acute PE. However, for hemodynamically unstable patients, inhaled pulmonary vasodilators (i.e. inhaled nitric oxide and epoprostenol) may be used.

- Percutaneous mechanical circulatory support devices (including VA-ECMO) are indicated for patients with refractory shock, i.e., not responding to thrombolysis/anticoagulation in patients with preload/afterload optimization and inotropic support.

- Surgical RVADs are rarely used for acute RV failure in patients with high-risk PE and are limited for patients who have failed medical management.

FUNDING

Dr Shore is currently supported by AHA grant ID 855105.

DISCLOSURE

The authors have nothing to disclose.

REFERENCES

1. Bělohlávek J, Dytrych V, Linhart A. Pulmonary embolism, part I: Epidemiology, risk factors and risk stratification, pathophysiology, clinical presentation, diagnosis and nonthrombotic pulmonary embolism. Exp Clin Cardiol 2013;18(2):129–38.

2. Haddad F, Doyle R, Murphy DJ, et al. Right Ventricular Function in Cardiovascular Disease, Part II. Circulation 2008;117(13):1717–31.

3. Konstam MA, Kiernan MS, Bernstein D, et al. Evaluation and Management of Right-Sided Heart Failure: A Scientific Statement From the American Heart Association. Circulation 2018;137(20):e578–622.

4. Sanz J, Sánchez-Quintana D, Bossone E, et al. Anatomy, Function, and Dysfunction of the Right Ventricle: JACC State-of-the-Art Review. J Am Coll Cardiol 2019;73(12):1463–82.

5. Matthews JC, McLaughlin V. Acute Right Ventricular Failure in the Setting of Acute Pulmonary Embolism or Chronic Pulmonary Hypertension: A Detailed Review of the Pathophysiology, Diagnosis, and Management. Curr Cardiol Rev 2008; 4(1):49–59.

6. Kapur NK, Esposito ML, Bader Y, et al. Mechanical Circulatory Support Devices for Acute Right Ventricular Failure. Circulation 2017;136(3):314–26.

7. Becattini C, Vedovati MC, Agnelli G. Prognostic Value of Troponins in Acute Pulmonary Embolism. Circulation 2007;116(4):427–33.

8. Becattini C, Casazza F, Forgione C, et al. Acute Pulmonary Embolism: External Validation of an Integrated Risk Stratification Model. Chest 2013; 144(5):1539–45.

9. Cavallazzi R, Nair A, Vasu T, et al. Natriuretic peptides in acute pulmonary embolism: a systematic review. Intensive Care Med 2008;34(12):2147–56.

10. Santos F, Albuquerque A, Ponciano A. Pulmonary embolism – EKG findings. Visual J Emerg Med 2021;25:101205.

11. Meinel FG, Nance JW, Schoepf UJ, et al. Predictive Value of Computed Tomography in Acute Pulmonary Embolism: Systematic Review and Meta-analysis. Am J Med 2015;128(7):747–59.e2.

12. Alerhand S, Sundaram T, Gottlieb M. What are the echocardiographic findings of acute right ventricular strain that suggest pulmonary embolism? Anaesth Crit Care Pain Med 2021;40(2):100852.

13. Management of PE. American College of Cardiology. Available at: https://www.acc.org/latest-in-cardiology/articles/2020/01/27/07/42/http%3a%2f%2fwww.acc.org%2flatest-in-cardiology%2farticles%2f2020%2f01%2f27%2f07%2f42%2fmanagement-of-pe. Accessed June 30, 2022.

14. Dalen JE, Alpert JS. Natural history of pulmonary embolism. Prog Cardiovasc Dis 1975;17(4):259–70.

15. Jaff MR, McMurtry MS, Archer SL, et al. Management of Massive and Submassive Pulmonary Embolism, Iliofemoral Deep Vein Thrombosis, and Chronic Thromboembolic Pulmonary Hypertension. Circulation 2011;123(16):1788–830.

16. Marik PE, Cavallazzi R. Does the central venous pressure predict fluid responsiveness? An updated meta-analysis and a plea for some common sense. Crit Care Med 2013;41(7):1774–81.

17. Ternacle J, Gallet R, Mekonso-Dessap A, et al. Diuretics in normotensive patients with acute pulmonary embolism and right ventricular dilatation. Circ J 2013;77(10):2612–8.

18. Schouver ED, Chiche O, Bouvier P, et al. Diuretics versus volume expansion in acute submassive pulmonary embolism. Arch Cardiovasc Dis 2017; 110(11):616–25.

19. Lim P, Delmas C, Sanchez O, et al. Diuretic vs. placebo in intermediate-risk acute pulmonary embolism: a randomized clinical trial. Eur Heart J Acute Cardiovasc Care 2022;11(1):2–9.

20. Ventetuolo CE, Klinger JR. Management of acute right ventricular failure in the intensive care unit. Ann Am Thorac Soc 2014;11(5):811–22.

21. Mercat A, Diehl JL, Meyer G, et al. Hemodynamic effects of fluid loading in acute massive pulmonary embolism. Crit Care Med 1999;27(3):540–4.

22. Rosenberger P, Shernan SK, Shekar PS, et al. Acute Hemodynamic Collapse After Induction of General Anesthesia for Emergent Pulmonary Embolectomy. Anesth Analg 2006;102(5):1311–5.

23. Stollings JL, Diedrich DA, Oyen LJ, et al. Rapid-sequence intubation: a review of the process and considerations when choosing medications. Ann Pharmacother 2014;48(1):62–76.

24. Ma KC, Chung A, Aronson KI, et al. Bronchoscopic intubation is an effective airway strategy in critically ill patients. J Crit Care 2017;38:92–6.

25. Schulman DS, Biondi JW, Matthay RA, et al. Effect of positive end-expiratory pressure on right ventricular performance: Importance of baseline right ventricular function. Am J Med 1988;84(1):57–67.

26. Zamanian RT, Haddad F, Doyle RL, et al. Management strategies for patients with pulmonary hypertension in the intensive care unit. Crit Care Med 2007;35(9):2037–50.

27. Disselkamp M, Adkins D, Pandey S, et al. Physiologic Approach to Mechanical Ventilation in Right Ventricular Failure. Annals ATS 2018;15(3):383–9.

28. Alviar CL, Miller PE, McAreavey D, et al. Positive Pressure Ventilation in the Cardiac Intensive Care Unit. J Am Coll Cardiol 2018;72(13):1532–53.

29. Ghignone M, Girling L, Prewitt RM. Volume expansion versus norepinephrine in treatment of a low cardiac output complicating an acute increase in right ventricular afterload in dogs. Anesthesiology 1984;60(2):132–5.

30. Gordon AC, Wang N, Walley KR, et al. The Cardiopulmonary Effects of Vasopressin Compared With Norepinephrine in Septic Shock. Chest 2012;142(3):593–605.

31. Rich S, Gubin S, Hart K. The Effects of Phenylephrine on Right Ventricular Performance in Patients with Pulmonary Hypertension. Chest 1990;98(5): 1102–6.

32. Tanaka H, Tajimi K, Matsumoto A, et al. Vasodilatory effects of milrinone on pulmonary vasculature in dogs with pulmonary hypertension due to pulmonary embolism: a comparison with those of dopamine and dobutamine. Clin Exp Pharmacol Physiol 1990;17(10):681–90.

33. 2019 ESC Guidelines for the diagnosis and management of acute pulmonary embolism developed in collaboration with the European Respiratory Society (ERS) | European Heart Journal | Oxford Academic. Available at: https://academic.oup.com/eurheartj/article/41/4/543/5556136. Accessed May 3, 2022.

34. Hirsh J, McDonald IG, Hale GA, et al. Comparison of the effects of streptokinase and heparin on the early rate of resolution of major pulmonary embolism. Can Med Assoc J 1971;104(6):488–91. passim.

35. Mlczoch J, Tucker A, Weir EK, et al. Platelet-Mediated Pulmonary Hypertension and Hypoxia during Pulmonary Microembolism: Reduction by Platelet Inhibition. Chest 1978;74(6):648–53.

36. Smith SB, Geske JB, Maguire JM, et al. Early Anticoagulation Is Associated With Reduced Mortality for Acute Pulmonary Embolism. Chest 2010;137(6):1382–90.

37. Douketis JD, Kearon C, Bates S, et al. Risk of fatal pulmonary embolism in patients with treated venous thromboembolism. JAMA 1998;279(6):458–62.

38. White RH. The Epidemiology of Venous Thromboembolism. Circulation 2003;107(23_suppl_1):I–4.

39. Tu T, Toma C, Tapson VF, et al. A Prospective, Single-Arm, Multicenter Trial of Catheter-Directed Mechanical Thrombectomy for Intermediate-Risk Acute Pulmonary Embolism: The FLARE Study. JACC Cardiovasc Interv 2019;12(9):859–69.

40. Baig MU, Bodle J. Thrombolytic Therapy. In: StatPearls. StatPearls Publishing; 2022. Available at: http://www.ncbi.nlm.nih.gov/books/NBK557411/. Accessed May 3, 2022.

41. Meyer G, Vicaut E, Danays T, et al. Fibrinolysis for Patients with Intermediate-Risk Pulmonary Embolism. N Engl J Med 2014;370(15):1402–11.

42. Daniels LB, Parker JA, Patel SR, et al. Relation of duration of symptoms with response to thrombolytic therapy in pulmonary embolism. Am J Cardiol 1997;80(2):184–8.

43. Chatterjee S, Chakraborty A, Weinberg I, et al. Thrombolysis for Pulmonary Embolism and Risk of All-Cause Mortality, Major Bleeding, and Intracranial Hemorrhage: A Meta-analysis. JAMA 2014;311(23):2414–21.

44. Marti C, John G, Konstantinides S, et al. Systemic thrombolytic therapy for acute pulmonary embolism: a systematic review and meta-analysis. Eur Heart J 2015;36(10):605–14.

45. Sharifi M, Bay C, Skrocki L, et al. Moderate Pulmonary Embolism Treated With Thrombolysis (from the "MOPETT" Trial). Am J Cardiol 2013;111(2):273–7.

46. Lyhne MD, Kline JA, Nielsen-Kudsk JE, et al. Pulmonary vasodilation in acute pulmonary embolism – a systematic review. Pulm Circ 2020;10(1). 2045894019899775.

47. Bhat T, Neuman A, Tantary M, et al. Inhaled nitric oxide in acute pulmonary embolism: a systematic review. Rev Cardiovasc Med 2015;16(1):1–8.

48. Khalid N, Rogers T, Shlofmitz E, et al. Adverse Events and Modes of Failure Related to Impella RP: Insights from the Manufacturer and User Facility Device Experience (MAUDE) Database. Cardiovasc Revascularization Med 2019;20(6):503–6.

49. Ravichandran AK, Baran DA, Stelling K, et al. Outcomes with the Tandem Protek Duo Dual-Lumen Percutaneous Right Ventricular Assist Device. Am Soc Artif Intern Organs J 2018;64(4):570–2.

50. Salna M, Garan AR, Kirtane AJ, et al. Novel percutaneous dual-lumen cannula-based right ventricular assist device provides effective support for refractory right ventricular failure after left ventricular assist device implantation. Interact Cardiovasc Thorac Surg 2020;30(4):499–506.

51. Eckman PM, Katz JN, El Banayosy A, et al. Veno-Arterial Extracorporeal Membrane Oxygenation for Cardiogenic Shock. Circulation 2019;140(24):2019–37.

52. Indications and Complications for VA-ECMO for Cardiac Failure. American College of Cardiology. Available at: https://www.acc.org/latest-in-cardiology/articles/2015/07/14/09/27/http%3a%2f%2fwww.acc.org%2flatest-in-cardiology%2farticles%2f2015%2f07%2f14%2f09%2f27%2findications-and-complications-for-va-ecmo-for-cardiac-failure. Accessed June 30, 2022.

53. Pasrija C, Kronfli A, George P, et al. Utilization of Veno-Arterial Extracorporeal Membrane Oxygenation for Massive Pulmonary Embolism. Ann Thorac Surg 2018;105(2):498–504. https://doi.org/10.1016/j.athoracsur.2017.08.033.

54. Karami M, Mandigers L, Miranda DDR, et al. Survival of patients with acute pulmonary embolism treated with venoarterial extracorporeal membrane oxygenation: A systematic review and meta-analysis. J Crit Care 2021;64:245–54.

55. Anderson MB, Goldstein J, Milano C, et al. Benefits of a novel percutaneous ventricular assist device for right heart failure: The prospective RECOVER RIGHT study of the Impella RP device. J Heart Lung Transplant 2015;34(12):1549–60.

56. Cheung AW, White CW, Davis MK, et al. Short-term mechanical circulatory support for recovery from acute right ventricular failure: clinical outcomes. J Heart Lung Transplant 2014;33(8):794–9.

57. Zuin M, Rigatelli G, Daggubati R, et al. Impella RP in hemodynamically unstable patients with acute pulmonary embolism. J Artif Organs 2020;23(2):105–12.

58. Kiernan MS, Krishnamurthy B, Kapur NK. Percutaneous right ventricular assist via the internal jugular vein in cardiogenic shock complicating an acute inferior myocardial infarction. J Invasive Cardiol 2010;22(2):E23–6.

59. Kapur NK, Paruchuri V, Korabathina R, et al. Effects of a percutaneous mechanical circulatory support device for medically refractory right ventricular failure. J Heart Lung Transplant 2011; 30(12):1360–7.

60. Samaranayake C, Garfield B, Seitler S, et al. Right ventricular assist devices for mechanical circulatory support in acute massive pulmonary embolism: a single centre experience. Eur Respir J 2021; 58(suppl 65). https://doi.org/10.1183/13993003. congress-2021.OA2594.

61. Arrigo M, Huber LC, Winnik S, et al. Right Ventricular Failure: Pathophysiology, Diagnosis and Treatment. Card Fail Rev 2019;5(3):140–6.

62. Nagpal AD, Singal RK, Arora RC, et al. Temporary Mechanical Circulatory Support in Cardiac Critical Care: A State of the Art Review and Algorithm for Device Selection. Can J Cardiol 2017;33(1):110–8.

63. Lahm T, McCaslin CA, Wozniak TC, et al. Medical and Surgical Treatment of Acute Right Ventricular Failure. J Am Coll Cardiol 2010;56(18):1435–46.

64. Bhalla A, Attaran R. Mechanical Circulatory Support to Treat Pulmonary Embolism: Venoarterial Extracorporeal Membrane Oxygenation and Right Ventricular Assist Devices. Tex Heart Inst J 2020; 47(3):202–6.

65. Berman M, Tsui S, Vuylsteke A, et al. Life-threatening Right Ventricular Failure in Pulmonary Hypertension: RVAD or ECMO? J Heart Lung Transplant 2008;27(10):1188–9.

66. DeFilippis EM. Mechanical Circulatory Support for Right Ventricular Failure. Published online November 19, 2021. Available at: https://www. cfrjournal.com/articles/mechanical-circulatory-support-right-ventricular-failure. Accessed June 19, 2022.

67. Salsano A, Sportelli E, Olivieri GM, et al. RVAD Support in the Setting of Submassive Pulmonary Embolism. J Extra Corpor Technol 2017;49(4):304–6.

68. Saif K, Kevane B, Áinle FN, et al. The role of the PERT team in 2021. Thrombosis Update 2022;6: 100092.

69. Chaudhury P, Gadre SK, Schneider E, et al. Impact of Multidisciplinary Pulmonary Embolism Response Team Availability on Management and Outcomes. Am J Cardiol 2019;124(9):1465–9.

70. Samaranayake CB, Craigie M, Kempny A, et al. Right heart strain assessment on CTPA following acute pulmonary embolism: Interobserver variability between expert radiologists and physicians. Respir Med 2022;200:106928.

Open Surgical Treatment of Acute and Chronic Pulmonary Embolism

Jonathan W. Haft, MD*, Gardner Yost, MD, MS

KEYWORDS

• Pulmonary embolism • Embolectomy • Thromboendarterectomy • Surgical

---

KEY POINTS

- Acute pulmonary embolism (PE) can cause hypoxia, right ventricular strain, and cardiovascular collapse.
- Acute PE with hemodynamic compromise can be treated with open surgical embolectomy.
- Chronic thromboembolic hypertension results from incomplete fibrinolysis of acute pulmonary emboli and presents as dyspnea and exertional intolerance.
- Chronic thromboembolism hypertension may be treated by open pulmonary endarterectomy, a procedure which, when performed at experienced centers, demonstrates excellent success rates.

INTRODUCTION

Acute pulmonary embolism (PE) is the third most common cause of death in the United States, after heart disease and cancer, and results in more than 630,000 symptomatic episodes yearly. 2.5 million Americans are diagnosed with deep vein thrombosis (DVT), and more than 90% of known PE is associated with lower extremity DVT.[1] Acute PE rarely necessitates open surgical intervention, excepting cases in which significant clot burden results in life-threatening hemodynamics, cor pulmonale, large mobile thrombi within the right atrium or ventricle, or a paradoxical embolus in transit.[2] However, surgical intervention is the treatment of choice for chronic PE leading to pulmonary hypertension.

Pathophysiology and Natural History of Deep Vein Thrombosis and Acute Pulmonary Embolism

The vast majority of PE is associated with lower extremity and pelvic DVT. These blood clots break off the vessel wall and travel through the right side of the heart into the pulmonary circulation.[3] This process, referred to as venous thromboembolism (VTE), produces a constellation of symptoms resulting from right ventricular (RV) pressure overload and ventilation to blood flow (V:Q) mismatch.[4] The causes of DVT include venous stasis, vein wall injury, and hypercoagulopathy, which together comprise Virchow triad. In hospitalized patients, immobilization is the most important cause of venous stasis, coupled with relative hypercoagulability associated with a postoperative state, infection, or malignancy. Genetic causes of hypercoagulability include deficiencies in antithrombin, Protein C or Protein S, and the Factor V Leiden mutation, among others.[5]

Embolic thrombi enter the pulmonary arteries through the right heart before lodging in the branch vessels. They are noted to predominantly affect the lower lobes because these receive a relatively larger fraction of the cardiac output. Once lodged within pulmonary arteries, the clot propagates because of stasis and activation of platelets and local endothelial cells. Activated platelets then release vasoconstrictors including

---

Cardiothoracic Surgery, University of Michigan, 1500 East Medical Center Drive 5144 CVC, Ann Arbor, MI 48109-5864, USA
* Corresponding author. 1500 East Medical Center Drive, Ann Arbor, MI 38109.
E-mail address: haft@med.umich.edu

Intervent Cardiol Clin 12 (2023) 339–347
https://doi.org/10.1016/j.iccl.2023.02.001
2211-7458/23/© 2023 Elsevier Inc. All rights reserved.

serotonin, thromboxane, and adenosine diphosphate, which superimpose further increases in pulmonary vascular resistance (PVR) with that generated by mechanical blockage of the pulmonary circulation by thrombus. The resulting redistribution of blood flow causes V:Q mismatch and hypoxemia.[6] The magnitude of the clot burden determines the reduction in cross-sectional area of the pulmonary arterial bed and, consequently, the significance of the hemodynamic compromise conferred by pulmonary emboli. Reduction in pulmonary arterial cross-sectional area drives an increase in PVR. Elevated PVR results in an increased RV afterload that may lead to ventricular dilation, ischemia, and dysfunction.[7] RV failure may result in tricuspid regurgitation, elevated CVP, and decreased LV preload, leading to decreased cardiac output, systemic hypotension, and organ congestion.

Untreated, the mortality of acute PE is 18% to 33% but is reduced to 8% if treated. Systemic anticoagulation permitting endogenous lysis of the emboli occurs over days to weeks in patients whose cardiopulmonary reserve is sufficient to survive the initial insult.[7]

Presentation and Diagnosis

Common symptoms of minor emboli include sudden anxiety, tachypnea, tachycardia, pleuritic chest pain, and cough. Submassive emboli present as the above symptoms with mild hemodynamic instability including relative hypotension and elevated CVP. Massive emboli present as the above with life-threatening hemodynamic instability. This is usually a result of occlusion of more than 50% of the pulmonary vasculature. Blood gases will reveal hypoxia and hypocarbia. Several diagnostic and imaging modalities are useful and necessary adjuncts in establishing a diagnosis. The electrocardiogram may demonstrate nonspecific T-wave and ST-segment changes. T-wave inversion in the anterior leads indicate ischemia inferiorly, typically a result of pressure overload. The classic pattern is S1Q3T3 (S wave on lead I, and Q and T waves in lead III). A chest radiograph may be helpful but should not delay a computed tomographic (CT) scan. A pleural effusion may be noted, and the absence of other causes of hypoxia (infiltrates, edema, or effusions) is helpful in arriving at a diagnosis. A CT pulmonary angiogram is considered the gold standard in the diagnosis of acute PE. This will show size and location of clot(s). The CT scan may provide additional information regarding ventricular dilation and the presence of other notable intracardiac pathology including thrombus in the right heart or in transit across a patent foramen ovale.[8] If imaging includes evaluations of the abdomen and pelvis, thrombi within the iliac system and inferior vena cava (IVC) may be identified. Other adjuncts include serum D-dimer levels, a fibrin degradation product, indicating fibrinolysis and is elevated in acute PE or DVT. Finally, echocardiography may be obtained.[9] Transthoracic echocardiography can demonstrate RV pressure overload, dysfunction, or distention and may reveal tricuspid regurgitation, paradoxical septal motion, or congestion of the IVC. Transesophageal echocardiography may identify thrombus in the main PA or central branches.

Treatment of Acute Pulmonary Embolism

The choice of treatment of acute PE is dictated by the identification of risk severity. High-risk patients are those demonstrating cardiogenic shock; intermediate-risk patients are those with signs of RV compromise as indicated by RV strain, RV dilation, S1Q3T3 EKG changes, troponin elevations, and others. Low-risk patients demonstrate none of the above signs. Open surgical treatment of PE with pulmonary embolectomy is a treatment modality only appropriate for a small group of patients who have acute PE—those classified as high risk and select patients classified as intermediate risk.[10] Specifically, patients who demonstrate hemodynamic compromise despite maximum medical treatment, including the use of thrombolytic therapy, warrant evaluation for surgery. These patients typically present with severely compromised pulmonary and cardiac function. Recent data demonstrates an operative mortality of 33% for patients undergoing open pulmonary embolectomy with cardiopulmonary bypass.[11] Survival is even worse for patients who require resuscitation with extracorporeal membrane oxygenation (ECMO) before embolectomy.[12] Management begins with cardiorespiratory stabilization followed by aggressive anticoagulation. Heparin prevents propagation of existing thrombi but does not cause clot lysis. Therapeutic anticoagulation permits fibrinolysis of the clot by endogenous factors over the period of days to weeks. ECMO may be used for cardiorespiratory support in the patient with profound hemodynamic compromise and may be continued until clot lysis results in reduced PVR.[13] Systemic thrombolysis with 100 mg of tissue plasminogen activator (tPA, alteplase) may be used to accelerate the lysis of thromboemboli when the diagnosis of PE has been confirmed and when the risk-to-benefit ratio is favorable. Thrombolytic therapy is associated with reduced all-cause mortality, reduced recurrent PE, and with improvement in RV function in hemodynamically unstable patients.[14] Thrombolytic therapy increases the risk of bleeding, most importantly, of intracranial hemorrhage, which occurs in up to 5% of patients.

Transcatheter thrombolysis

Transcatheter thrombolysis is an emerging procedure for treating massive and submassive PE.[15] Several therapies are available for transcatheter thrombolysis, including flow-directed lytic infusion, suction devices, and ultrasonic devices. According to the pulmonary embolism response to fragmentation, embolectomy, and catheter thrombolysis (PERFECT) trial, typical treatment with fibrinolytic is delivery of 0.5 to 2.0 mg of tissue plasminogen activator per hour for a total dose of 20 to 28 mg.[16] The ultrasound accelerated thrombolysis of pulmonary embolism (ULTIMA) study randomized the use of ultrasonic-assisted thrombolysis catheters, which combined fibrinolytic therapy with high-frequency, low-intensity ultrasound waves against anticoagulation alone demonstrated a short-term hemodynamic improvement without significant difference in 90-day mortality.[17]

Acute pulmonary embolectomy

Indications.   Primary indications for acute pulmonary embolectomy remain highly individualized and guided by the experience and judgement of the operating surgeon. This is, at least partially, because the acute nature of presentation with PE makes a true clinical trial challenging, if not impossible, to conduct.[18] Guidelines from the American Heart Association and the European Society of Cardiology suggest that indications for surgical therapy include massive or submassive PE with cardiovascular collapse, RV dysfunction and troponin leak in the absence of shock, and when catheter-based treatments have failed or are unavailable and systemic lytic therapy is contraindicated. Contraindications to thrombolytic therapy include a history of intracranial hemorrhage, intracranial malignancy, mass, or aneurysm; cerebral vascular accident within the past 3 months, recent major surgery. Large highly mobile thrombi in transit within the right atrium or ventricle require urgent surgical treatment, along with trapped thrombi within a patent foramen ovale (paradoxical embolus in transit).[14,19]

Surgical technique.   A midline sternotomy is performed followed by central cannulation. Many of these patients are profoundly hemodynamically unstable, and this can be exacerbated by induction of general anesthesia. The surgical team must be prepared to proceed at a rapid pace if necessary. Peripheral cannulation may be an acceptable alternative and may afford a more expedient initiation of bypass. The bilateral groins should be prepared for rapid vascular access and possible ECMO initiation before the induction of anesthesia. Cardioplegia and cross-clamping are required if a patent foramen ovale (PFO) repair or other intracardiac procedure, such as clot retrieval, is planned on the left side of the heart, so as to avoid air embolization.

The main PA is incised longitudinally 1 to 2 cm distal to the pulmonic valve; the conal branches of the RCA may be used as landmarks for this arteriotomy. Suction and forceps are used to remove emboli. If thrombus is located in the left PA, this incision may be extended toward the pericardial reflection on the left pulmonary artery. If thrombus is located in the right PA beyond the bifurcation, a separate incision in the right PA can be made longitudinally between the superior vena cava (SVC) and aorta.

If necessary, additional maneuvers may be performed to further remove the clot. The pleural spaces may be opened and the lungs compressed to expel distal clot. Retrograde perfusion may be used through the pulmonary veins to flush clot in a retrograde direction; this requires aortic cross-clamping and cardioplegia. Once complete, the pulmonary arteriotomies are closed. Patching is rarely necessary.[7,13,20]

Postoperative management following acute pulmonary embolectomy is often challenging due to the critical nature of the disease process. Postoperative complications include RV dysfunction, cardiogenic shock, hypoxia, and bleeding; all of which must be treated aggressively, recognizing the inherent need for balanced volume resuscitation and RV support. There is typically a low threshold to initiate extracorporeal life support. Inotropes and prolonged mechanical ventilatory support are frequently required.[7,21] Anticoagulation should be initiated in the postoperative period once chest tube output is acceptable. The patient should remain on oral anticoagulation for at least 6 months, or longer in the cases of recurrent or unprovoked PE. The risk of recurrent PE with appropriate postoperative anticoagulation is less than 5%. Several studies have demonstrated that direct oral anticoagulants are noninferior to warfarin in the treatment of VTE.[22]

Outcomes.   Surgical pulmonary embolectomy was first attempted by Trendelenberg in 1908 at which time the mortality was close to 100%. Following the advent of cardiopulmonary bypass and use of heparin, Cooley performed the first successful surgical embolectomy in 1961.[12,23] The published description of operative mortality for patients undergoing pulmonary embolectomy varies considerably with early reports demonstrating mortality as high as 78% and an average of 33% for patients undergoing pulmonary embolectomy with cardiopulmonary bypass and 56% for those undergoing embolectomy without cardiopulmonary bypass, which is referred to as the "classic," or "Trendelenberg" approach. Importantly, rates of mortality have been steadily improving over time with recent reports demonstrating in-hospital mortality in the rage of 5% to 6%.[8,10,11,13]

Owing to the acute and critical nature of the disease process, a randomized clinical trial comparing surgical to medical treatment of acute PE has not been performed, and there are few studies comparing the approaches in a nonrandomized fashion. Gulba and colleagues[24] demonstrated a mortality of 23% in patients treated with surgical embolectomy versus 33% in patients treated with thrombolysis. A study by Meneveau and colleagues[25] examined patients who had failed thrombolysis. Of these, 14 underwent surgical intervention and 26 had repeat thrombolysis. Rates of mortality were 7% and 38%, respectively. Generalization using these studies must be tempered by the knowledge that they are small, retrospective, and lack controls.

Interestingly, several studies have reported good outcomes after surgical embolectomy with liberalized indications. Specifically, recognizing that the presence of RV strain and hemodynamic compromise is a strong predictor for postoperative RV failure, some centers have proceeded to surgical embolectomy for patients with echocardiographic evidence of moderate-to-severe RV strain but without hemodynamic compromise. These studies have demonstrated mortality in the range of 6% to 10%[22,26]

Complications associated with surgical embolectomy are common. The most frequent complication is heart failure followed by pulmonary hemorrhage secondary to reperfusion of an ischemic or infarcted lung, pulmonary failure, and neurologic damage. Recurrent PE after embolectomy is a feared complication, which is responsible for significant mortality. Meneaveau and colleagues[27] demonstrated that recurrent PE was responsible for one-third of postembolectomy deaths; however, IVC filter insertion after surgical embolectomy remains somewhat controversial. Nonetheless, current American College of Chest Physicians guidelines recommend the placement of an IVC filter if anticoagulation is contraindicated or if there is recurrent embolism despite anticoagulation.[9]

Chronic Thromboembolic Disease

Background. Chronic thromboembolic pulmonary hypertension (CTEPH) is thought to develop in 0.5% to 5% of patients with acute PE because of incomplete thrombolysis.[26] This amounts to 5.7 cases per million population, a number that is increasing and is expected to continue to increase.[28] The prevalence of CTEPH has increased in recent decades due to increased awareness and improved imaging, including the use of CT pulmonary angiography, which generates slices on the order of 0.5 to 1 mm and useful multiplane reconstruction.[29]

The basic pathogenesis of CTEPH is incomplete lysis of pulmonary emboli. This may occur from lack of anticoagulant treatment or an associated hypercoagulable disorder. Fibrin within the clot progressively becomes cross-linked and organized, leading to incorporation and endothelialization. In some cases, partial lysis results in partial recanalization leaving webs or stenoses.[30]

The phenomenon of CTEPH results only partially from the mechanical obstruction to the segmental branches of the pulmonary vasculature. Blood flow is redirected into the relatively unobstructed segments. These hyperperfused segments undergo pulmonary vascular changes, similar to Eisenmenger syndrome, from excessive pulmonary blood flow. These pulmonary vascular changes include medial hypertrophy, vasoconstriction, and the formation of plexiform lesions and thromboses. This constellation of findings results in progressive pulmonary hypertension and RV failure in the absence of recurrent pulmonary emboli.[31]

Presentation and Diagnosis

The most common presenting symptom of CTEPH is exertional dyspnea, often out of proportion to clinical examination. Patients may also complain of chest pain, hemoptysis, and peripheral edema. CTEPH is defined as a mean PA pressures greater than 25 mm Hg more than 6 months after PE, PVR greater than 3 Woods units, and pulmonary capillary wedge pressure less than 15 mm Hg. Approximately 25% of patients will not be aware of a history of PE.[32] A chest radiograph may demonstrate right heart enlargement and dilated pulmonary arteries. Echocardiogram will identify pulmonary

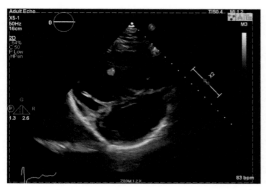

Fig. 1. Echocardiographic image demonstrating 2 chamber view of a patient with CTEPH with resultant RV dilation and septal shift, which results in a "D"-shaped left ventricle.

hypertension using the tricuspid regurgitation jet velocity, and may note chronic sequelae of pulmonary hypertension such as morphologic changes to the right ventricle resulting in dilation and the appearance of a D-shaped left ventricle (Fig. 1). In the absence of other causes of pulmonary hypertension (left heart disease, advanced pulmonary parenchymal pathology), a VQ scan is indicated. A normal result excludes the diagnosis of CTEPH but the presence of any mismatched ventilation:perfusion defects warrants further testing. Pulmonary angiography remains the gold standard for the diagnosis of CTEPH and will clarify the burden of disease and surgical accessibility.[30] (Fig. 2) Some patients will have significant symptoms but no evidence of pulmonary hypertension at rest. In this case, invasive cardiopulmonary exercise testing may demonstrate features consistent with symptomatic

chronic PE including a rapid increase in PA pressures with exercise, blunted cardiac output response, and increase in CO_2 from dead space ventilation.

Pulmonary endarterectomy for CTEPH

Indications. Pulmonary endarterectomy (PEA) by experienced surgeons is the standard treatment in symptomatic patients with CTEPH with surgically accessible disease. They should be evaluated at a center with significant experience in the procedure, its diagnostic imaging, and perioperative care.

The following criteria should be met.

- WHO class II-IV symptoms
- Preoperative PVR >300 dynes $\times$ seconds $\times$ cm^{-5}
- Surgically accessible thrombi in the main, left/right, lobar, segmental, or subsegmental arteries, as determined by providers with substantial experience in PEA
- Comorbidities and functional status that are not prohibitive for surgical correction and recovery

There may be some patients that do not meet these criteria but are determined to have surgically accessible disease in the absence of pulmonary hypertension, referred to as chronic thromboembolic disease (CTED). These patients should undergo invasive cardiopulmonary exercise testing to confirm that exertional intolerance is related to CTED and not to underlying pulmonary disease or deconditioning.

The level of the obstruction in the pulmonary arteries is described according to the Jamieson classification.

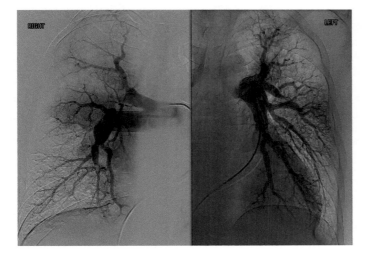

Fig. 2. Pulmonary angiogram for the right and left pulmonary arteries demonstrating significant and diffuse stenosis bilaterally.

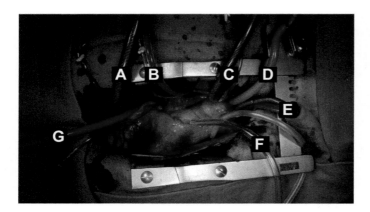

Fig. 3. The standard cannulation for pulmonary thromboendarterectomy before cross-clamp placement. (*A*) IVC cannula, (*B*) left ventricular vent placed in the right superior pulmonary vein, (*C*) SVC cannula, (*D*) SVC snare, (*E*) Aortic cannula, (*F*) cardioplegia tubing, not yet connected to cardioplegia cannula, and (*G*) IVC snare.

- *Type I.* Organized obstructing clot in the main branch PA
- *Type II.* Organized thrombus in the lobar branches; most frequent (40%–70%)
- *Type III.* Obstructive disease at the segmental level
- *Type IV.* Disease limited to the subsegmental branches

Surgical technique

The patient is positioned supine with the arms tucked, and a radial arterial line, central line, and Foley catheter are placed after the induction of anesthesia. The procedure is performed via median sternotomy using central aortic and bicaval venous cannulation with caval snares. The left ventricle is vented through the right superior pulmonary vein and aortic root (**Fig. 3**). Aortic cross-clamping and standard cardioplegia are used. Deep hypothermic circulatory arrest (18°C) is mandatory to eliminate back-bleeding from what is typically robust bronchial collateral flow. This permits visualization of the distal pulmonary branches during the endarterectomy. The pulmonary artery is dissected off the SVC. The SVC is mobilized circumferentially to the azygous vein. The aorta is cross-clamped and cardioplegia administered to achieve diastolic arrest. Collapse of the ascending aorta below the clamp facilitates exposure of the right PA. The cava are snared. The SVC is retracted laterally and the aorta medially to expose the right PA, which is opened longitudinally beyond the orifice of the upper lobe trunk. The endarterectomy is then begun on the right side by entering the proper plane between organized thrombus and normal intima (**Fig. 4**). The key element of the PTE is identification of the correct endarterectomy plane within the pulmonary artery. This can be challenging due to obfuscation of places

by chronic disease, back bleeding, and difficult surgical anatomy. The proper plane is indicated by the presence of a pearly white layer and ideally is carried around the vessel for 360°.

Using the "hand-over-hand" technique, gentle traction on the endarterectomy specimen while sweeping away the wall of the pulmonary artery often permits separation of the organized thrombus and vessel wall.[29] In many cases, the removal of several separate specimens is necessary to achieve a complete endarterectomy (**Fig. 5**). Intervals of circulatory arrest of up to 20 minutes with 10 minutes of reperfusion are used to permit the endarterectomy to be carried

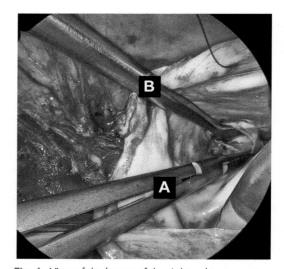

Fig. 4. View of the lumen of the right pulmonary artery (RPA), with demonstration of identification of the endarterectomy plane. In this image the grasping instrument (Labeled "*A*") is pulling the endarterectomy specimen away from the vessel wall, which is being retracted (with retractor labeled "*B*") toward the top of the image.

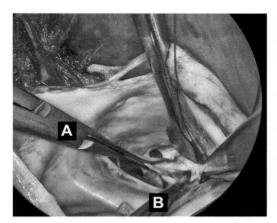

Fig. 5. View of an endarterectomy specimen being removed from an upper lobe branch of the RPA. In this image, the grasping instrument (Labeled "A") is being used to provide tension on the endarterectomy specimen while the suction instrument (Labeled "B"), is being used to coax the vessel wall away free from the specimen.

into each subsegmental branch individually. The right PA is closed with fine running polypropylene suture during a period of reperfusion (Fig. 6). The left PA is approached through an incision from the distal main PA carried into the left PA to the pericardial reflection, and the process is repeated. Once complete, the cross-clamp is removed and the patient is rewarmed while the left pulmonary arteriotomy is closed. The patient separated from cardiopulmonary bypass, often with very little inotropic support. Fig. 7 demonstrates the specimens removed from a single patient arranged to indicate their locations within the pulmonary arteries.

Postoperative care and complications
In the immediate postoperative period, patients should remain mechanically ventilated with relatively higher tidal volumes to encourage recruitment of the lower lobes that may receive a disproportionate amount of the pulmonary blood flow. Anticoagulation must be initiated as soon as it is safe from a perioperative bleeding perspective. These patients will require anticoagulation for the remainder of their lives. Despite RV dysfunction preoperatively, after a successful endarterectomy, significant RV support is rarely required. Pulmonary hemorrhage is a rare but life-threatening complication resulting from full thickness injury, often at the subsegmental level. Emergent bronchoscopy to identify the side of hemorrhage, followed by insertion of a double lumen endotracheal tube to isolate to nonhemorrhaging lung. Catheter-based embolization is typically required, often with ECMO support. Reperfusion injury occurs in approximately 10% of patients and is associated with desaturation and presence of edema-like fluid in the airways. Treatment is supportive with careful management of ventilation, and aggressive diuresis.

Outcomes
Successful resection of occlusive disease results in significant hemodynamic and symptomatic improvements including exercise capacity and functional status in the majority of patients.[32,33]

In experienced centers, in-hospital mortality has been reported to be as low as 2.2%.[34] A recent prospective registry using data from 27 centers and 679 patients demonstrates 1, 2, and 3-year survivals of 93%, 89%, and 88% respectively. This study identified several correlates for worsened postoperative survival including, but not limited to, poor functional status, increased right atrial pressure, and postoperative pulmonary hypertension.[35] Inadequate reduction in PVR is the biggest risk factor for mortality. A single-center study demonstrated mortality as high as 10.3% in patients with residual pulmonary hypertension after PTE compared with 0.9% in patients without.[36] Long-term

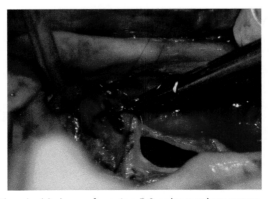

Fig. 6. The RPA is closed with a double layer of running 5-0 polypropylene suture.

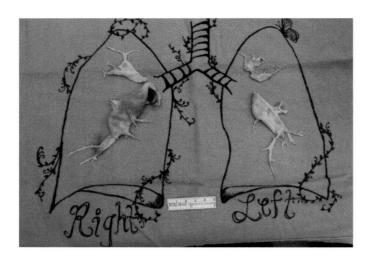

Fig. 7. The endarterectomy specimens are placed on a surgical towel in anatomic position.

survival following pulmonary endarterectomy is excellent, with preservation in the reduction of pulmonary artery pressures.[37]

CLINICS CARE POINTS

- Diagnosis of PE is best obtained via a pulmonary embolism protocol CT with contrast. The extent of pulmonary and hemodynamic compromise is key to determining next steps in management.

- Open surgical or catheter based embolectomy may be considered in patients with acute PE and hemodynamic compromise if systemic thrombolysis has failed or is contraindicated.

- Pumonary endarterectomy for chronic thromboembolic pulmonary hyptersion should be considered in symptomatic patients with surgically accessible disease who are appropriate surgical candidates and who have pulmonary vascular resistance in excess of 300 Dynes x seconds x cm^-5.

- Surgical treatment of CTEPH in specialized centers demonstrates exellent survival, sympomatic relief, and improvements in pulmonary artery pressures.

DISCLOSURE

The authors have no disclosures.

DECLARATION OF INTERESTS

The authors declare that they have no known competing financial interests or personal relationships that could have appeared to influence the work reported in this paper.

REFERENCES

1. LeVarge B, Wright C, Rodriguez-Lopez J. Surgical management of acute and chronic pulmonary embolism. Clin Chest Med 2018;39:659–67.
2. Yavuz S, Toktas F, Goncu T, et al. Surgical embolectomy for acute massive pulmonary embolism. Int J Clin Exp Med 2014;7:5362–75.
3. Carson JL, Kelley MA, Duff A, et al. The clinical course of pulmonary embolism. N Engl J Med 1992;326:1240–5.
4. Hoagland PM. Massive pulmonary embolism. In: Goldhaber SZ, editor. Pulmonary embolism and deep venous thrombosis. Philadelphia: Saunders; 1985. p. 179–208.
5. Alpert JS, Dalen JE. Epidemiology and natural history of venous thromboembolism. Prog Cardiovasc Dis 1994;36:417–22.
6. Smulders YM. Pathophysiology and treatment of haemodynamic instability in acute pulmonary embolism: the pivotal role of pulmonary vasoconstriction. Cardiovasc Res 2000;48:23–33.
7. Licha CRM, McCurdy CM, Maldonaldo SM, et al. Current management of acute pulmonary embolism. Ann Thorac Cardiovasc Surg 2020;26:65–71.
8. Choong CK, Calvert PA, Falter F, et al. Life-threatening impending paradoxical embolus caught 'red-handed': successful management by multidisciplinary team approach. J Thorac Cardiovasc Surg 2008;136:527–8.
9. Torbicki A, Perrier A, Konstantinides S, et al. Guidelines ESCCP Guidelines on the diagnosis and management of acute pulmonary embolism: the task force for the diagnosis and management of acute pulmonary embolism of the European Society of Cardiology (ESC). Eur Heart J 2008;29:2276–315.
10. Kadner A, Schmidli J, Schonhoff F, et al. Excellent outcome after surgical treatment of massive

pulmonary embolism in critically ill patients. J Thorac Cardiovasc Surg 2008;136:448–51.

11. Yalamanchili K, Fleisher AG, Lehrman SG, et al. Open pulmonary embolectomy for treatment of major pulmonary embolism. Ann Thorac Surg 2004;77:819–23.

12. Cooley DA, Beall AC, Alexander JK. Acute massive pulmonary embolism: successful surgical treatment using temporary cardiopulmonary bypass. JAMA 1961;177(5):283–6.

13. Leacche M, Unic D, Goldhaber SZ, et al. Modern surgical treatment of massive pulmonary embolism: results in 47 consecutive patients after rapid diagnosis and aggressive surgical approach. J Thorac Cardiovasc Surg 2005;129:1018–23.

14. Jaff MR, McMurtry MS, Archer SL, et al. Management of massive and submassive pulmonary embolism, iliofemoral deep vein thrombosis, and chronic thromboembolic pulmonary hypertension: a scientific statement from the American Heart Association. Circulation 2011;123:1788–830.

15. Meyer G, Koning R, Sors H. Transvenous catheter embolectomy. Semin Vasc Med 2001;1(2):247–52.

16. Kucher N, Boekstegers P, Muller OJ, et al. Randomized, controlled trial of ultrasound-assisted catheter-directed thrombolysis for acute intermediate-risk pulmonary embolism. Circulation 2014;129:479–86.

17. Kuo WT, Banerjee A, Kim PS, et al. Pulmonary embolism response to fragmentation, embolectomy, and catheter thrombolysis (PERFECT): initial results from a prospective multicenter registry. Chest 2015;148:667–73.

18. Sanchez O, Planquette B, Meyer G. Management of massive and submassive pulmonary embolism: focus on recent randomized trials. Curr Opin Pulm Med 2014;20(5):393–9.

19. Konstantinides SV. 2014 ESC guidelines on the diagnosis and management of acute pulmonary embolism. Eur Heart J 2014;35:3145–6.

20. Akay TH, Sezgin A, Ozkan S, et al. Successful surgical treatment of massive pulmonary embolism after coronary bypass surgery. Tex Heart Inst J 2006;33:498–500.

21. Elassal AA, Jabbad HH, Al-Ibrahim KI. Rescue surgical pulmonary embolectomy for acute massive pulmonary embolism. J Egypt Soc Cardio Thorac Surg 2016;24:166–72.

22. Eldredge JB, Spyropoulos AC. Direct oral anticoagulants in the treatment of pulmonary embolism. Curr Med Res Opin 2018;34(1):131–40.

23. He C, Von Segesser LK, Kappetein PA, et al. Acute pulmonary embolectomy. Eur J Cardio Thorac Surg 2013;43(6):1087–95.

24. Gulba DC, Schmid C, Borst HG, et al. Medical compared with surgical treatment for massive pulmonary embolism. Lancet 1994;343:576–7.

25. Meneveau N, Seronde MF, Blonde MC, et al. Management of unsuccessful thrombolysis in acute massive pulmonary embolism. Chest 2006;129:1043–50.

26. Aklog L, Williams CS, Byrne JG, et al. Acute pulmonary embolectomy: a contemporary approach. Circulation 2002;105:1416–9.

27. Meneveau N. Therapy for acute high-risk pulmonary embolism: thrombolytic therapy and embolectomy. Curr Opin Cardiol 2010;25(6):560–7.

28. Poli D, Miniati M. The incidence of recurrent venous thromboembolism and chronic thromboembolic pulmonary hypertension following a first episode of pulmonary embolism. Curr Opin Pulm Med 2011;17(5):392–7.

29. Heit JA, Spencer FA, White RH. The epidemiology of venous thromboembolism. J Thromb Thrombolysis 2016;41:3–14.

30. Papamatheakis DG, Poch DS, Fernandes TM, et al. Chronic thromboembolic pulmonary hypertension: JACC focus seminar. J Am Coll Cardiol 2020;76(18):2155–69.

31. de Perrot M, Donahoe L. Pulmonary Thromboendarterectomy: how I teach it. Ann Thorac Surg 2018;106(4):945–50.

32. Saouti N, Morshuis WJ, Heijmen RH, et al. Long-term outcome after pulmonary endarterectomy for chronic thromboembolic pulmonary hypertension. Eur J Cardio Thorac Surg 2009;35:947–52.

33. Pepke-Zaba J, Delcroix M, Lang I, et al. Chronic thromboembolic pulmonary hypertension (CTEPH): results from an international prospective registry. Circulation 2011;124. 1973-2198.

34. Madani MM, Auger WR, Pretrorius V, et al. Pulmonary endarterectomy: recent changes in a single institution's experience of more than 2,700 patients. Ann Thorac Surg 2012;94:97–103.

35. Delcroix M, Lang I, Pepke-Zaba J, et al. Long-term outcome of patients with chronic thromboembolic pulmonary hypertension; results from an international prospective registry. Circulation 2016;133:859–71.

36. Mayer E, Jenkins D, Lindner J, et al. Surgical management and outcome of patients with chronic thromboembolic pulmonary hypertension: results from an international prospective registry. J Thorac Cardiovasc Surg 2011;141:702–10.

37. Pesavento R, Filippi L, Palla A, et al. Impact of residual pulmonary obstruction on the long-term outcome of patients with pulmonary embolism. Eur Respir J 2017;49:160.

Cardiopulmonary Exercise Testing, Rehabilitation, and Exercise Training in Postpulmonary Embolism

Naga Dharmavaram, MD[a], Amir Esmaeeli, MD[a],
Kurt Jacobson, MD[a], Yevgeniy Brailovsky, DO, MSc[b],
Farhan Raza, MD[a],*

KEYWORDS

• Pulmonary embolism • Postpulmonary embolism syndrome • Cardiopulmonary exercise test
• Exercise training • Rehabilitation

KEY POINTS

• Exercise intolerance and functional impairments 3 to 6 months after an acute pulmonary embolism (PE) are common and should be investigated with cardiopulmonary exercise test (CPET).
• If significant CPET abnormalities are detected (reduced peak VO_2, abnormal V_E/VCO_2), further testing should be performed, which includes ventilation perfusion scan for pulmonary vascular occlusion from residual thrombus and echocardiogram for pulmonary hypertension and right heart failure.
• Exercise training and rehabilitation should be discussed and prescribed.
• It remains unclear if treatments beyond anticoagulation, catheter-directed therapies, and thrombolytics affect functional impairments at 3 to 6 months post-PE.

INTRODUCTION

Long-term exercise intolerance and functional limitations are common after an episode of acute pulmonary embolism (PE), despite 3 to 6 months of anticoagulation.[1] These persistent symptoms are reported in more than half of the patients with acute PE and are referred as "post-PE syndrome."[2] Although these functional limitations can occur from persistent pulmonary vascular occlusion or pulmonary vascular remodeling,[3] significant deconditioning can be a major contributing factor.[4] Herein, the authors review the role of exercise testing to elucidate the mechanisms of exercise limitations to guide next steps in management and exercise training for musculoskeletal deconditioning.

POST-PULMONARY EMBOLISM EXERCISE IMPAIRMENT

After an episode of acute PE, anticoagulation for at least 3 months is recommended for most patients with provoked PE (due to an identifiable reversible risk factor, eg, surgery, estrogen use, trauma, and immobility).[5–7] A prolonged and indefinite anticoagulation should be considered in select cases (unprovoked PE, persistent risk factor, recurrent PE). Most of the clinical improvement and acute clot resolution occurs in the

[a] Division of Cardiology, Department of Medicine, University of Wisconsin-Madison, Hospitals and Clinics, 600 Highland Avenue CSC-E5/582B, Madison, WI 53792, USA; [b] Division of Cardiology, Department of Medicine, Jefferson Heart Institute-Sidney Kimmel School of Medicine, Thomas Jefferson University, 111 South 11th Street, Philadelphia, PA 19107, USA
* Corresponding author. University of Wisconsin-Madison, Hospitals and Clinics, 600 Highland Avenue CSC-E5/582B, Madison, WI 53792.
E-mail address: fraza@medicine.wisc.edu

Intervent Cardiol Clin 12 (2023) 349–365
https://doi.org/10.1016/j.iccl.2023.02.002
2211-7458/23/© 2023 Elsevier Inc. All rights reserved.

first 3 months,[8,9] and the optimal time to assess residual exercise impairment is 3 to 6 months after the acute PE episode.[4,10,11]

As indicated in **Fig. 1**, there are 3 possible sequalae after treatment of acute PE after 3 to 6 months of anticoagulation. Although most patients have resolution of clot, nearly 30% have residual pulmonary vascular obstruction from chronic thromboembolic disease. Among these patients, some have no resting pulmonary hypertension (chronic thromboembolic disease [CTED]), and others develop chronic thromboembolic pulmonary hypertension (CTEPH, nearly 4% of all patients post-PE).[2,12] As indicated in **Fig. 2**, persistent functional limitations can occur from varying and overlapping causes and should be quantified with exercise testing.[13,14] Additional ancillary testing should be considered with ventilation perfusion (VQ) scan and echocardiogram to assess for persistent perfusion defects, pulmonary hypertension (PH), and right ventricular dysfunction.[4,10,11]

Quality-of-Life Surveys

A variety of quality-of-life (QoL) questionnaires are available to assess functional impairments in patients after acute PE. Besides generic QoL questionnaires, such as the 36-Item Short Form Health Survey (SF-36) and Kansas City Cardiomyopathy Questionnaire (KCCQ), there are PE-specific questionnaires, such as the Pulmonary Embolism Quality of Life Questionnaire (PEmb-QoL). The PEmb-QoL questionnaire is a reliable instrument to assess QoL after acute PE.[15] It includes 9 questions and assesses 6 domains: frequency of complaints, activities of daily living limitations, work-related problems, social limitations, intensity of complaints, and emotional complaints. Higher scores indicate a worse QoL.

The FOCUS (Follow-Up after Acute Pulmonary Embolism) study is a prospective, multi-center trial that followed-up patients for 2 years after the event of an acute PE. The trial assessed QoL measures via the PEmb-QoL questionnaire at 3 and 12 months following acute PE. At the 3-month mark, patients could be divided into tertiles, with 34.4% feeling worse than baseline, 29.9% feeling the same, and 26% feeling better than baseline. At the 12-month mark, 55.4% felt better than baseline, whereas 20.3% had complete resolution of problems/symptoms. The data from the trial showed that at both time points, worse QoL was associated with female sex, elevated body mass index (BMI), and preexisting cardiopulmonary disease.[16]

The ELOPE (Prospective Evaluation of Long-term Outcomes After Pulmonary Embolism) study, examined post-PE effects on dyspnea, QoL, and exercise capacity after treatment with warfarin. The study found that most patients had improvement in these dimensions over 1 year, with the greatest improvement manifesting in the first 3 months after treatment.[9] It also found that female sex, elevated BMI, and poor exercise-capacity measured at 1 month post-PE (defined by percent-predicted oxygen consumption VO_2 less than 80% on cardiopulmonary exercise) was associated with worse outcomes.[17]

A similar study by Josien and colleagues reported that in 109 post-PE patients QoL (per SF-36 and PEmb-QoL surveys at a median follow-up of 25 months post-PE) was reduced and comparable to patients with acute myocardial infarction the previous year.[18] More importantly, the study suggested that higher thrombus load did not seem to affect QoL on the long-term.

Cardiopulmonary Exercise Test

In addition to QoL surveys, a symptom-limited cardiopulmonary exercise testing (CPET) is the best tool to assess functional impairments in various cardiopulmonary diseases.[19–23] It provides diagnostic value in discriminating multi-system contributions in multifactorial dyspnea and prognostic value to determine clinical outcomes.[19,21,24]

A. *CPET metrics*: the methodology and measurements of CPET are described in the ATS/ACCP statement[25] and other detailed reviews.[17,19,26,27] Herein, we present a more simplified stepwise approach as a practical guide to interpreting CPET. (1) *Peak VO_2*: peak VO_2, adjusted for weight (mL/Kg/min) and reported as percentage predicted (based on age and sex), indicates the maximal exercise capacity. Peak VO_2 less than 80% of predicted indicates exercise intolerance in post-PE patients.[23,28] (2) *Respiratory exchange ratio (RER)*: peak exercise RER (carbon dioxide output: VCO_2 to VO_2 ratio), greater than or equal to 1.1 indicates a good effort, RER less than 1.0 indicates a poor, whereas an RER 1.0 to 1.1 indicates a fair effort.[17] An RER less than 1.1 suggests deconditioning and inability to cross anaerobic threshold (AT), albeit coronary artery disease (CAD), and chronic obstructive pulmonary disease (COPD) can also be a major limiting factor.[17,19,25,26] (3) *Gas exchange, V_E/VCO_2*: linking minute

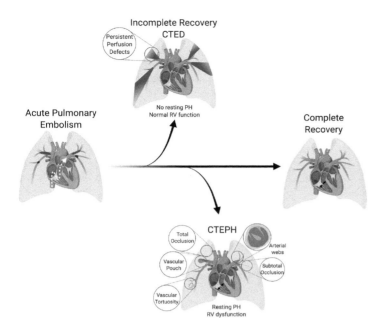

Fig. 1. Sequalae after treatment of acute pulmonary embolism with 3 to 6 months of anticoagulation. CTED, chronic thromboembolic disease; CTEPH, chronic thromboembolic pulmonary hypertension; PH, pulmonary hypertension; RV, right ventricle. Figure created using Biorender.com.

ventilation (V_E) to VCO_2 results in matching ventilation-to-perfusion response to exercise and is defined as ventilatory efficiency.[17] V_E/VCO_2 reflects efficiency of alveolar-capillary interface, chemoreceptor sensitivity, and acid-base balance. With exercise, there is improved VQ matching and reduction in V_E/VCO_2 till AT is achieved. There is an increase in V_E/VCO_2 after AT due to metabolic acidosis and hyperventilation. Similar to V_E/VCO_2, other metrics of gas exchange improve with exercise: $PETCO_2$ (partial pressure of end-tidal carbon dioxide) increases, and V_D/V_T (physiologic dead-space fraction) decreases.[27] Abnormal V_E/VCO_2 correlates with symptoms and disease severity in cardiopulmonary diseases with V_E/VCO_2 greater than 35 considered a high-risk

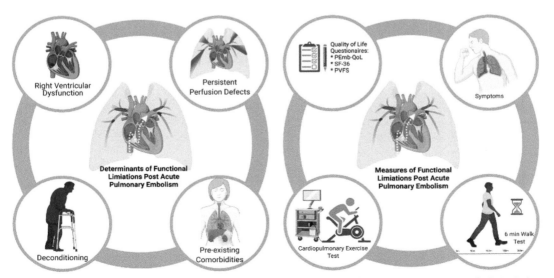

Fig. 2. Postpulmonary embolism functional limitations: quantifying and determining causes. PEmb-QoL, Pulmonary Embolism Quality of Life Questionnaire; PVFS, post-venous thromboembolism functional status; SF-36, 36-Item Short Form Health Survey. Figure created using Biorender.com.

feature.[17,19,22,25,27,29,30] Zhai and colleagues reported that V_E/VCO_2 (mean value) is worse in CTEPH (51), versus a comparable pulmonary arterial hypertension (PAH) cohort (44) with similar peak VO_2.[31] McCabe and colleagues reported that nadir V_E/VCO_2 at AT (mean value) can differentiate normal subjects (27) from CTED (37) and CTEPH (46).[13] These studies indicate the additional burden of poor gas exchange and breathlessness from residual thrombus, even in the absence of pulmonary vascular disease. (4) *Breathing Reserve (BR)*: BR corresponds to ventilatory (lung parenchymal) reserve at peak exercise and is traditionally defined as the percentage of MVV (maximal ventilatory volume = FEV1 x 35–40) achieved at peak exercise ([$V_E$max/ MVV] x 100%).[25] A breathing reserve less than 15% to 20% suggests pulmonary disease as a primary cause of dyspnea. However, there is significant reported variance in normal value for BR, and some studies suggesting that BR less than 15% to 20% can underestimate true ventilatory limitation of COPD even with relatively low-intensity exercise.[32] (5) O_2 *pulse*: oxygen pulse (O_2 pulse = VO_2/heart rate) is a reasonable surrogate of stroke volume and indicates cardiac response to exercise (eg, right ventricular limitation to exercise in a post-PE patient). However, O_2 pulse also depends on arteriovenous oxygen difference (O_2 extraction), and different thresholds have not been extensively validated. In a study of patients with heart failure with reduced ejection fraction (HFrEF) (n = 209), Lavie and colleagues reported that an O2 pulse greater than or equal to 10 mL/beat predicted event-free survival on a follow-up of 40 months.[33] (6) *Heart rate*: a normal exercise response requires a nearly 2.2-fold increase in heart rate, and the augmentation of heart rate from rest to exercise is referred as heart rate reserve (HRR).[34] Inability to achieve greater than or equal to 80% of HRR or greater than or equal to 80% of age-predicted maximal heart rate (220-age) indicates chronotropic incompetence (CI).[34,35] CI is identified as a major contributory factor to chronic cardiopulmonary diseases, including post-PE (ELOPE study).[23,34,35] It remains unclear if CI reflects peripheral muscle deconditioning or reduced cardiac beta-receptor sensitivity.[36] However, cardiac rehabilitation has been shown to improve CI in patients with CAD,[37] and 6-minute walk distance in patients with heart failure.[38] Recovery of heart rate after exercise also indicates good cardiovascular health and is defined as decrease in heart rate from peak exercise to 2 minutes of recovery of less than 42 beats per minute.[34,39] (8) *Miscellaneous*: peripheral oxygen desaturation (SpO_2) with exercise is a sign of pulmonary vascular disease such as CTEPH or thromboembolic disease without PH such as CTED.[23,31] Exercise oscillatory ventilation has been described in postcapillary PH, presumed due to stimulation of pulmonary J-receptors from increase in left-heart filling pressures, but not reported in PAH or thromboembolic disease.[19] Lastly, VO_2 kinetics reveal significant patterns of cardiopulmonary limitations in PH and heart failure,[19,20,40] which are beyond the scope of the current review.

B. *CPET modality: Treadmill versus ergometer*: CPET can be performed with a treadmill or cycle ergometer (upright or recumbent in most noninvasive laboratories). In comparison to cycle ergometer, treadmill CPET results in a higher peak VO_2 due to increased muscle mass recruitment.[25,26] However, cycle ergometer provides significant benefits that include higher safety, less noise, ease of ramp protocol, and blood gas collection.[25,26]

Regarding impact of exercise modality on V_E/VCO_2, Valli and colleagues reported on 13 patients with severe PAH (mean pulmonary artery pressure = 65 mm Hg) undergoing treadmill and ergometer CPETs 24 to 48 hours apart.[41] The study reported a higher V_E/VCO_2 ratio at anaerobic threshold with treadmill (56) versus ergometer (45). Although the sample size was small, the investigators suggested that treadmill test provided a more accurate depiction of VQ abnormalities and disease severity. Based on this study, a treadmill CPET may be better suited for post-PE patients undergoing CPET to identify physiologic dead-space from vascular occlusions.

C. *CPET in cardiopulmonary diseases and post-PE state*: CPET provides significant prognostic information in different cardiopulmonary diseases, as summarized in Table 1. More importantly, it can identify burden of cardiopulmonary versus peripheral muscular limitations and guide management steps after 3 to 6 months of anticoagulation in a post-PE patient. In the

Table 1			
Major cardiopulmonary exercise studies in different cardiopulmonary diseases			
Study	**Details**	**Modality**	**Major Findings**
HFrEF Mancini DM, et al,[21] 1991	Prospective N = 122, mean age = 50 y, 15% women	Treadmill	Three subgroups: 1. Peak $VO_2 > 14$ mL/Kg/min (n = 52) had 94% 1-y survival 2. Peak $VO_2 < 14$ mL/Kg/min (n = 27) and not transplant candidates had 47% 1-y survival 3. Peak $VO_2 < 14$ mL/Kg/min (n = 35) and awaiting transplant had 70% 1-y survival
HFrEF Osman AF, et al,[44] 2000	Prospective N = 225, mean age = 54 y, 20% women	Treadmill	Peak VO_2 mL/Kg/min <19 per lean body mass is superior to peak $VO_2 < 14$ in predicting outcomes Percent fat = 25.9% in the cohort, and 37% subjects had BMI $\geq$30 kg/m^2
HFrEF Arena R, et al,[29] 2007	Prospective N = 448, mean age = 57 y, 21% women	Treadmill	Based on V_E/VCO_2, 4 groups were defined: (i) $\leq$29, (ii) 30-35.9, (iii) 36-44.9, (iv) $\geq$45.0 and had respectively predictive event-free survival at 2 y: 97%, 85%, 72%, and 44%
PAH Yasunobu, et al,[45] 2005	Retrospective N = 52 (control = 9), mean age = 44 y, 86% women	Cycle ergometer	Four PAH subgroups per peak VO_2 %-predicted (mild: 65%-79%; moderate: 50%-64%; severe: 35%-49%; very severe: 35%), control = 93% 1. V_E/VCO_2 ratio at AT significantly higher in all PAH subgroups (37, 42, 45, 67), control = 27 2. $PETCO_2$ (mm Hg) at AT was lower in all PAH subgroups (33, 28, 26, and 18), control = 42

(continued on next page)

Table 1
(continued)

Study	Details	Modality	Major Findings
PAH Sun, et al,[46] 2001	Retrospective N = 53 (20 controls), mean age = 42 y, 88% women	Cycle ergometer	V_E/VCO_2 slope was significantly higher in PAH subjects (47) compared with controls (25) Peak VO_2 (mL/kg/min) was significantly lower in PAH (12) compared with controls (30)
HFpEF Dhakal, et al,[47] 2015	Prospective N = 48 (controls = 24), mean age = 63 y, women = 60%	Invasive CPET with upright cycle ergometer	Peak VO_2 (mL/kg/min) = 13.9 (27.0 in controls) Impaired peripheral oxygen extraction (C[a-v]O_2 = 11.5 mL/dL vs 13.3 mL/dL in controls) and reduced peak heart rate (121 vs 148 in controls)
CTEPH Zhai, et al,[31] 2011	Retrospective N = 50 (PAH = 77), mean age = 60 y, women = 46%	Cycle ergometer	Worse dead space ventilation in CTEPH: V_E/VCO_2 slope = 51 (44 in PAH), despite similar peak VO_2 (mL/kg/min) 13.8 in CTEPH, vs 14.5 in PAH.
Post-PE ELOPE study Kahn SR, et al,[23] 2017	Prospective N = 100, mean age = 50 y, 43% women	Cycle ergometer	46.5% patients had peak VO_2 <80% predicted (n = 86 pts completed 1-y follow-up) Reduced peak VO_2 attributed to deconditioning; not predicted by residual thrombus on repeat imaging.[42]
Post-PE Albaghdadi Mazen S, et al,[43] 2018	Prospective N = 20, mean age = 57 y, 40% women	Cycle ergometer	12/20 (60%) with peak VO_2 <80% at 6-mo. Deconditioning suggested as predominant cause of persistent dyspnea

Abbreviations: AT, anaerobic threshold; BMI, body mass index; C[a-v]O2, arteriovenous oxygen concentration difference; CTEPH, chronic thromboembolic pulmonary hypertension; HFpEF, heart failure with preserved ejection fraction; HFrEF, heart failure with reduced ejection fraction; PAH, pulmonary arterial hypertension; PETCO2, partial pressure of end-tidal carbon dioxide; VE/VCO2, minute ventilation to carbon dioxide production; VO2, oxygen consumption.

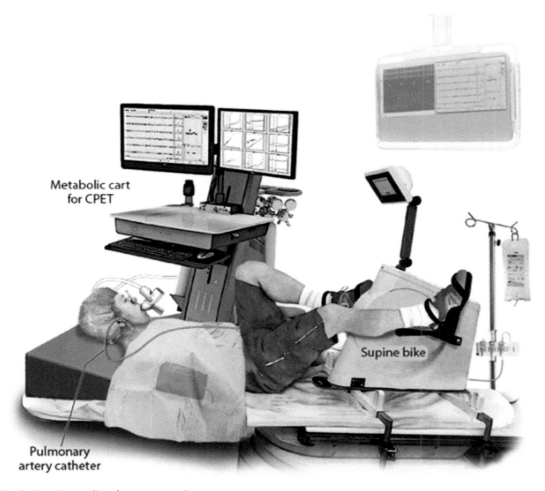

Metabolic cart
for CPET

Supine bike

Pulmonary
artery catheter

Fig. 3. Invasive cardiopulmonary exercise test.

ELOPE study,[23] reduced exercise capacity was associated with male sex, elevated BMI, and history of smoking. Most (87.5%) of those with diminished exercise capacity were due to physical deconditioning; however, a significant minority (12.5%) were due to ventilatory defects. Subsequent imaging analysis revealed no correlation of residual perfusion defects with reduced peak VO_2.[42] These findings suggest that physical deconditioning is the main cause for residual exercise impairment in post-PE patients. Similar prospective study by Albaghdadi and colleagues in 20 post-PE patients suggests reduced peak VO_2 in 60% patients, predominantly due to deconditioning.[43]

D. *Invasive CPET:* in subjects with exercise impairment and CPET abnormalities, with suspected CTED or CTEPH, an invasive CPET can confirm the diagnosis and guide PAH vasodilator therapies. A cycle ergometer is used for invasive CPET studies either in an upright, supine, or recumbent position.

The detailed methods are described by expert centers.[48–52] Briefly, a right internal jugular venous access for a pulmonary arterial catheter and a right radial cannula for arterial monitoring is placed. Ramp protocol on a cycle ergometer is used for rest-to-exercise invasive CPET study, along with a metabolic cart (Figs. 3 and 4). Pressure flow (direct Fick cardiac output) measurements are acquired during different stages of exercise. A lactate level is checked at peak exercise to confirm elevated level and adequacy of effort. Based on

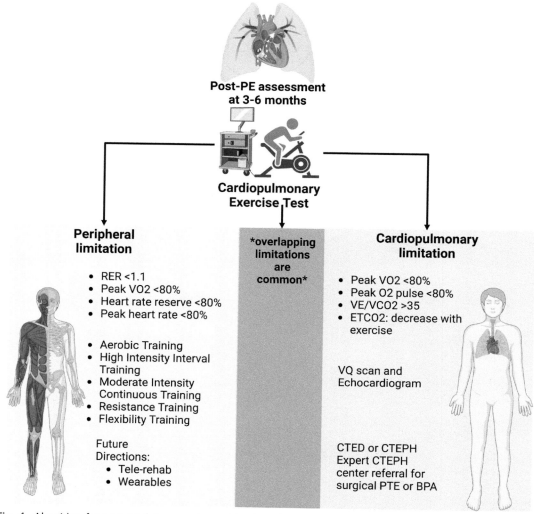

Fig. 4. Algorithm for post-PE follow-up. *, combination of peripheral limitation and cardiopulmonary limitation. BPA, balloon pulmonary angioplasty; CTED, chronic thromboembolic disease; CTEPH, chronic thromboembolic pulmonary hypertension; ETCO₂, end-tidal carbon dioxide pressure; O₂ pulse, oxygen pulse (VO₂/heart rate); PE, pulmonary embolism; RER, respiratory exchange ratio; V_E/VCO_2, minute ventilation to carbon dioxide output ratio; VO₂, oxygen consumption; VQ, ventilation-perfusion. Figure created using Biorender.com.

established criteria for exercise PH,[4,49,53,54] the hemodynamic diagnosis of post-PE patients is confirmed as CTED or CTEPH. These criteria include mean pulmonary artery pressure/cardiac output slope greater than or equal to 3 mm Hg/L/min[49] and peak exercise transpulmonary resistance greater than or equal to 3 mm Hg/L/min[53].

Six-Minute Walk Test
Six-minute walk test (6MWT) is a simple and reproducible tool to assess functional limitations.[55–57] It has been extensively used in clinical

trials, and its correlation with CPET metrics and NYHA class has been reported.[58] Miyamoto and colleagues reported a study of 43 PAH patients undergoing 6MWT and CPET. Walk distance in NYHA classes (2/3/4) was ~440, 320, and 100 m. Median 6MWT of 332 m predicted clinical outcomes on 5-year follow-up. 6MWT correlated modestly with cardiac output (r = 0.48, P < .05) and total pulmonary resistance (r = −0.49, P < .05) and strongly with peak VO₂ (r = 0.70, P < .001), and V_E/VCO_2 slope (r = −0.66, P < .001). 6MWT is a useful tool in centers that lack CPET facilities.

EXERCISE TRAINING IN CARDIOPULMONARY DISEASE

Peripheral muscle deconditioning is present in nearly half post-PE patients.[23,59] These limitations are reported even after receiving thrombolytics (PEITHO trial),[60] whereas more studies are needed to assess long-term limitations in patients receiving catheter-directed thrombolytics for acute PE.[61–64] To address the deconditioning, pulmonary and cardiac rehabilitation have been a mainstay in the treatment of PAH, HFrEF, HFpEF (heart failure with preserved ejection fraction), and COPD in helping increase exercise capacity and various aspects of psychosomatic health.[65–67] These chronic conditions produce skeletal muscle alterations, detraining, and deconditioning.[68] Further, Lowe and colleagues have shown that a reduction in exercise capacity in the setting of PH has been associated with depression and anxiety.[69]

In post-PE patients, early participation in exercise and structured rehabilitation programs have been found safe and effective in multiple studies (Table 2).[70–73] In some studies, exercise regimen was started as early as 1-month post-PE.[72,80] Although in-person pulmonary rehabilitation has been used in most studies, remote home-based regimen has been reported to be efficacious for post-PE patients,[72] similar to CAD and heart failure.[77,81] Hence for post-PE patients, the American Physical Therapy Association has published guidelines for physical therapist to implement exercise regimen after an episode of thromboembolic disease.[82]

Exercise Goals

The goals of a cardiac rehabilitation program are to assess a patient's baseline ability and limitations, develop an exercise prescription, observe the patient's response to that prescription, and encourage long-term participation in regular unsupervised exercise. Through these 4 goals, the goal of increasing the patient's cardiorespiratory fitness can be achieved.[83] Additional components of a successful rehabilitation program include psychosocial support, nutritional counseling, weight management, and education regarding diet and medications adherence. All these nonexercise goals further bolster the efficacy of a rehabilitation program[84] and improve patient's cardiorespiratory fitness.

For the best balance of recruiting large muscle groups while still avoiding a higher risk of physical injury, low-impact, aerobic exercises are preferred for a rehabilitation program. Examples include walking, jogging, cycling, rowing, or machine stair climbing.[85] It is important, however, to individualize the exercise regimen to the individual as to promote maximum compliance and reduce risk of injury. To engage the individual, several different types of exercise routines have been studied.

Exercise Modalities

A. *Aerobic exercise training*: aerobic exercise training has been the mainstay of cardiac rehabilitation. Saltin and colleagues demonstrated in 1968 the benefits of exercise in the Dallas Bed Rest and Exercise study,[86] and it was Braunwald, Sarnoff, Sonnenblick, Hellerstein, and Naughton, among others who helped lay the foundation for the present-day cardiac rehabilitation program.[87,88] Twenty percent reduction in all-cause mortality has been observed for each metabolic equivalent improvement in fitness in those with cardiovascular disease.[89]

B. *Moderate intensity continuous training (MICT)*: based on current consensus, MICT consists of aerobic activity that falls within the 60% of maximal heart rate or a 12 to 13 on the Borg scale.[90] MICT has been reported to achieve an increase in the peak VO_2.[90–92]

C. *High-intensity interval training (HIIT)*: recent research has shown that higher intensity exercise leads to greater improvements in peak VO_2 than moderate- or low-intensity exercise. Taylor and colleagues reported a 10% increase in peak VO_2 with HIIT versus a 4% with MICT in patients with CAD.[93] HIIT has been shown to significantly improve respiratory muscle function, ventilatory drive, lung diffusion, and alveolar-capillary conductance, which all contributed to a higher peak VO_2.[94–96] Peripheral vascular adaptations with HIIT include increases in mean blood flow through increases in shear stress stimulus and upregulation of vasodilatory mechanisms, leading to improved endothelial function and flow-mediated dilation, eventually leading to increased peak VO_2.[97–100] Lastly, improved oxidative capacity and mitochondrial adaptations in skeletal muscles enhance O_2 extraction and utilization.[101–103]

D. *Resistance training*: resistance training is an important and safe component of rehabilitation.[104,105] Ozaki and colleagues reported that older patients with a low baseline peak VO_2 (<25 mL kg^{-1} min^{-1})

Table 2
Major studies on rehabilitation and structured exercise programs in postpulmonary embolism and other cardiopulmonary diseases

Study Name	Disease	Type of Exercise Regimen	Modality of Exercise	Frequency of Exercise	Duration of Exercise	Major Outcomes/Findings
PeRehab Study Haukeland-Parker, et al,[70] 2021	Post-PE	Outpatient rehabilitation vs usual care	Interval and resistance training	2x per wk	8 wk	Ongoing trial n = 190, 1:1 randomization
Pulmonary rehabilitation post-PE and cardiac MRI Gleditsch, et al,[71] 2022	Post-PE	Outpatient rehabilitation vs usual care	Supervised resistance and endurance training	2x per wk	8 wk	n = 26, significant improvement in "Shortness of Breath Questionnaire" (median 15–8) and reduction in right ventricular mass (49–44 g)
Physiotherapist-guided home-based exercise Rolving et al,[72] 2020	Post-PE	Home-based vs usual care	Variable (patient-preferred exercise modality)	3x per wk	8 wk	n = 140 with 1:1 randomization and exercise regimen 1–3 mo post-PE. Exercise was safe Improvement in incremental shuttle walk test on 6-mo follow-up: 104 vs 78 m (P = .27)
Pulmonary rehabilitation post-PE Nopp et al,[73] 2020	Post-PE	Single-arm intervention	Cycle ergometer, inspiratory muscle training	3x per wk	6 wk	n = 22, rehabilitation started 19 wk post-PE 6MWD improved by 49.4 m on completion
Fox et al,[74] 2011	PAH, CTEPH	6 wk HIIT and 6 wk MICT	Treadmill, cycling, step climbing, resistance training	24 1-h sessions	12 wk	Increase in 6MWD by 32 m and VO_2Max by 1.1 mL kg^{-1} min^{-1}. No serious adverse events

Study	Population	Comparison	Modality	Frequency	Duration	Outcome
HF-ACTION O'Connor et al,[75] 2009	Chronic heart failure	Exercise training vs usual care	Cycle or treadmill	3x per wk	12 wk	11% reduction in all-cause mortality/hospitalizations and a 13% reduction in cardiovascular mortality or heart failure hospitalizations
SAINTEX-CAD Conraads et al,[76] 2015	Coronary artery disease	In-person rehab	HIIT vs MICT	3x per wk	12 wk	Both interval and continuous training improve VO$_2$Max (22.7 vs 20.3 mL kg^{-1} min^{-1}) at 12 wk and this is sustained at 1 y
REMOTE-CR Maddison et al,[77] 2019	Coronary heart disease	Telerehab vs in-person rehab	Individualized to each participant	3x per wk	12 wk	Peak VO$_2$ was noninferior; telerehab less sedentary at 24 wk; per capita program delivery and medication costs lower for telerehab
Yoga-CaRe Prabhakaran et al,[78] 2020	Acute myocardial infarction	Yoga vs standard care	Yoga	13 sessions in 12 wk	12 wk	Yoga improved self-rated health and return to preinfarct activities
Ries et al,[79] 2005	COPD	Walking	Pulmonary rehabilitation	Twice daily for 30 min	8 wk	Pulmonary rehab in COPD associated with increased exercise tolerance (1.5 METS vs 0.6 METS)

Abbreviations: 6MWD, 6-minute walk distance; COPD, chronic obstructive pulmonary disease; CTEPH, chronic thromboembolic pulmonary hypertension; HIIT, high-intensity interval training; LVEDD, left ventricular end diastolic volume; MICT, moderate-intensity continuous training; PAH, pulmonary arterial hypertension; PE, pulmonary embolism; VO$_2$Max, maximal oxygen consumption.

benefited more from resistance training than those with a higher baseline peak VO_2 (>32 mL kg^{-1} min^{-1}).[106] Hence, sicker patients stand to benefit the most from resistance training.

E. *Flexibility training: Yoga and Tai Chi:* Yoga-CaRe study evaluated the benefit of yoga in cardiac rehabilitation for patients with recent acute myocardial infarction. Although it did not have enough power to show a statistically significant difference in major adverse cardiovascular events, it improved self-rated health and return to preinfarct activities.[78] Liu and colleagues studied Tai chi (another low-impact and low-intensity exercise), and found it to improve aerobic endurance and psychosocial well-being in those with CAD.[107]

Exercise Dose: Frequency, Intensity, and Duration

A rehabilitation program will typically include 3 times a week session for 8 to 12 weeks. A typical rehabilitation session starts with a 5- to 10-minute warm up, followed by 20 to 45 minutes of aerobic activity, and concluded by a 5- to 10-minute cool down. The intensity of exercise ranges from 40% to 85% of peak VO_2 (55%–90% of maximal heart rate [HR] = 220-age). The intensity of exercise based on maximal heart rate is characterized as follows:

a Light exercise: <60% of max HR
b Moderate exercise: 60% to 79% of max HR
c Heavy exercise: ≥80% of max HR

Another measure of exertion that is commonly used in rehabilitation programs is the "rating of perceived exertion" (RPE) on the Borg scale. The scale is measured from 6 to 20 and an RPE of 12 to 13 is perceived to be "somewhat hard," which should correlate to 60% of the peak VO2, and an RPE of 16 is perceived to be "hard-to-very hard," which correlates to 85% of peak VO2.[108] Based on these studies, an individualized light-to-moderate exercise regimen should be routinely prescribed in patients with functional impairments due to muscle deconditioning at 3 months post-PE; this is supported by the 2019 combined guidelines by the European Society of Cardiology and the European Respiratory Society.[109]

Synergy Between Exercise and Medical Interventions

Post-PE cardiopulmonary limitations include residual clot, PAH, right heart dysfunction, and previously undiagnosed left heart disease (CAD, HFpEF). It is essential to have a synergy of prompt management of cardiopulmonary limitations, as the exercise therapies are used.

Although studying the individualized benefit of exercise regimen versus cardiopulmonary intervention is difficult, the exercise regimen is proved to improve the overall health of any patient with a cardiopulmonary comorbidity.[110,111]

Future Directions: Telerehabilitation and Wearables

Technology-assisted delivery methods (telerehabilitation) can overcome significant barriers of health care accessibility and lower costs. REMOTE-CR trial of 162 patients with CAD, delivered remotely monitored telerehabilitation (n = 82) and center-based rehabilitation (n = 80).[112] Telerehabilitation delivery (vs in-person rehabilitation) was equally effective (peak VO_2 at 12-week: 30.5 vs 29.4 mL/Kg/min), with significantly lower costs.[77] Future studies are needed to validate these findings in patients after acute PE. With the advent of wearable health monitoring devices such as the Apple Watch, WHOOP, Garmin, and Fitbit, there has been a renewed interest in incorporating them into the cardiac rehabilitation world. In addition, given the relative equivalence of remote versus center-based delivery of rehabilitation services, these devices could be a paradigm shift in the concept of cardiac rehabilitation.[113,114] Given the COVID-19 pandemic and the costs associated with traveling to a center-based program, wearable-assisted home programs could further enhance participation and long-term compliance.

SUMMARY

After 3 to 6 months of anticoagulation for acute PE, residual functional impairments and exercise intolerance are present in more than half of the patients. Although residual thromboembolic burden exists in nearly one-third cases, deconditioning contributes to exercise impairment in nearly all these patients. Different modality and delivery methods of structured exercise regimen should be used for long-term improvements in exercise capacity and quality of life.

CLINICS CARE POINTS

- In assessing a patient at 3-months after an acute PE episode, assess residual exercise intolerance with history and consider a cardiopulmonary exercise test to objectify.

- If persistent dyspnea or CPET abnormalities exist, consider a VQ scan and echocardiogram.
- For peripheral muscle deconditioning, prescribe structured exercise regimen.

ACKNOWLEDGMENTS

None.

REFERENCES

1. Klok FA, Tijmensen JE, Haeck MLA, et al. Persistent dyspnea complaints at long-term follow-up after an episode of acute pulmonary embolism: Results of a questionnaire. Eur J Intern Med 2008;19(8):625–9.
2. Klok FA, van der Hulle T, den Exter PL, et al. The post-PE syndrome: A new concept for chronic complications of pulmonary embolism. Blood Rev 2014;28(6):221–6.
3. Nijkeuter M, Hovens MMC, Davidson BL, et al. Resolution of thromboemboli in patients with acute pulmonary embolism: A systematic review. Chest 2006;129(1):192–7.
4. Morris TA, Timothy M, Fernandes RC. How we do it: evaluation of dyspnea and exercise intolerance after acute pulmonary embolism. Chest 2022. S0012-3692(22)01215-01216.
5. Prediletto R, Paoletti P, Fornai E, et al. Natural course of treated pulmonary embolism. Evaluation by perfusion lung scintigraphy, gas exchange, and chest roentgenogram. Chest 1990;97(3):554–61.
6. Baglin T, Bauer K, Douketis J, et al. Duration of anticoagulant therapy after a first episode of an unprovoked pulmonary embolus or deep vein thrombosis: Guidance from the SSC of the ISTH. J Thromb Haemost 2012;10(4):698–702.
7. Kearon C, Akl EA, Comerota AJ, et al. Antithrombotic therapy for VTE disease: Antithrombotic therapy and prevention of thrombosis, 9th ed: American College of Chest Physicians evidence-based clinical practice guidelines. Chest 2012; 141(2 SUPPL):e419S–96S.
8. Van Es J, Douma RA, Kamphuisen PW, et al. Clot resolution after 3 weeks of anticoagulant treatment for pulmonary embolism: Comparison of computed tomography and perfusion scintigraphy. J Thromb Haemost 2013;11(4):679–85.
9. Kahn SR, Akaberi A, Granton JT, et al. Quality of Life, Dyspnea, and Functional Exercise Capacity Following a First Episode of Pulmonary Embolism: Results of the ELOPE Cohort Study. Am J Med 2017;130(8):990.
10. Boon GJAM, Bogaard HJ, Klok FA. Essential aspects of the follow-up after acute pulmonary embolism: An illustrated review. Res Pract Thromb Haemost 2020;4(6):958–68.
11. Pugliese SC, Kawut SM. The post-pulmonary embolism syndrome: Real or ruse? Ann Am Thorac Soc 2019;16(7):811–4.
12. Pengo V, Lensing AWA, Prins MH, et al. Incidence of Chronic Thromboembolic Pulmonary Hypertension after Pulmonary Embolism. N Engl J Med 2004;350(22):2257–64.
13. Mccabe C, Deboeck G, Harvey I, et al. Inefficient exercise gas exchange identifies pulmonary hypertension in chronic thromboembolic obstruction following pulmonary embolism. Thromb Res 2013;132(6):659–65.
14. Topilsky Y, Hayes CL, Khanna AD, et al. Cardiopulmonary exercise test in patients with subacute pulmonary emboli. Heart & Lung J Acute Crit Care 2012;41(2):125–36.
15. Klok FA, Cohn DM, Middeldorp S, et al. Quality of life after pulmonary embolism: validation of the PEmb-QoL Questionnaire. J Thromb Haemost 2010;8(3):523–32.
16. Valerio L, Barco S, Jankowski M, et al. Quality of life 3 and 12 months following acute pulmonary embolism: analysis from a prospective multicenter cohort study. Chest 2021;159(6):2428–38.
17. Milani RV, Lavie CJ, Mehra MR, et al. Understanding the basics of cardiopulmonary exercise testing. Mayo Clin Proc 2006;81(12):1603–11.
18. Josien vE, Paul L den, Kaptein A, et al. Quality of life after pulmonary embolism as assessed with SF-36 and PEmb-QoL. Thromb Res 2013;132(5): 500–5.
19. Malhotra R, Bakken K, D'Elia E, et al. Cardiopulmonary Exercise Testing in Heart Failure. JACC Hear Fail 2016. https://doi.org/10.1016/j.jchf.2016.03.022.
20. Chatterjee NA, Murphy RM, Malhotra R, et al. Prolonged mean vo2 response time in systolic heart failure an indicator of impaired right ventricular-pulmonary vascular function. Circ Hear Fail 2013; 6(3):499–507.
21. Mancini DM, Eisen H, Kussmaul W, et al. Value of peak exercise oxygen consumption for optimal timing of cardiac transplantation in ambulatory patients with heart failure. Circulation 1991;83(3): 778–86.
22. Weatherald J, Farina S, Bruno N, et al. Cardiopulmonary exercise testing in pulmonary hypertension. Annals of the American Thoracic Society 2017;14(Supplement_1):S84–92.
23. Kahn SR, Hirsch AM, Akaberi A, et al. Functional and Exercise Limitations After a First Episode of Pulmonary Embolism: Results of the ELOPE

Prospective Cohort Study. Chest 2017;151(5):1058–68.

24. Popovic D, Arena R, Guazzi M. A flattening oxygen consumption trajectory phenotypes disease severity and poor prognosis in patients with heart failure with reduced, mid-range, and preserved ejection fraction. Eur J Heart Fail 2018;20(7):1115–24.

25. Weisman IM, Weisman IM, Marciniuk D, et al. ATS/ACCP Statement on cardiopulmonary exercise testing. Am J Respir Crit Care Med 2003;167(2):211–77.

26. Mezzani A. Cardiopulmonary exercise testing: Basics of methodology and measurements. Ann Am Thorac Soc 2017;14:S3–11.

27. Arena R, Guazzi M, Myers J, et al. Cardiopulmonary exercise testing in the assessment of pulmonary hypertension. Expert Rev Respir Med 2011. https://doi.org/10.1586/ers.11.4.

28. Kahn SR, Hirsch A, Beddaoui M, et al. Post-Pulmonary Embolism Syndrome" after a First Episode of PE: Results of the E.L.O.P.E. Study. Blood 2015;126(23):650.

29. Arena R, Myers J, Abella J, et al. Development of a ventilatory classification system in patients with heart failure. Circulation 2007;115(18):2410–7.

30. Al JWET, Weatherald J, Philipenko B, et al. Ventilatory efficiency in pulmonary vascular diseases. Eur Respir Rev 2021;30(161):200214.

31. Zhai Z, Murphy K, Tighe H, et al. Differences in ventilatory inefficiency between pulmonary arterial hypertension and chronic thromboembolic pulmonary hypertension. Chest 2011;140(5):1284–91.

32. O'Donnell DE, Elbehairy AF, Faisal A, et al. Exertional dyspnoea in COPD: The clinical utility of cardiopulmonary exercise testing. Eur Respir Rev 2016;25(141):333–47.

33. Lavie CJ, Milani RV, Mehra MR. Peak exercise oxygen pulse and prognosis in chronic heart failure. Am J Cardiol 2004;93(5):588–93.

34. Brubaker PH, Kitzman DW. Chronotropic incompetence: Causes, consequences, and management. Circulation 2011;123(9):1010–20.

35. Zweerink A, van der Lingen ALCJ, Handoko ML, et al. Chronotropic Incompetence in Chronic Heart Failure. Circ Heart Fail 2018;11(8):e004969.

36. Sarma S, Stoller D, Hendrix J, et al. Mechanisms of chronotropic incompetence in heart failure with preserved ejection fraction. Circ Hear Fail 2020;1–9. https://doi.org/10.1161/CIRCHEARTFAILURE.119.006331.

37. Pimenta T, Rocha JA. Cardiac rehabilitation and improvement of chronotropic incompetence: Is it the exercise or just the beta blockers? Rev Port Cardiol 2021;40(12):947–53.

38. Mentz RJ, Whellan DJ, Reeves GR, et al. Rehabilitation Intervention in Older Patients With Acute Heart Failure With Preserved Versus Reduced Ejection Fraction. JACC Hear Fail 2021;9(10):747–57.

39. Cole CR, Foody JAM, Blackstone EH, et al. Heart rate recovery after submaximal exercise testing as a predictor of mortality in a cardiovascularly healthy cohort. Ann Intern Med 2000;132(7):552–5.

40. Bailey CS, Wooster LT, Buswell M, et al. Post-Exercise Oxygen Uptake Recovery Delay: A Novel Index of Impaired Cardiac Reserve Capacity in Heart Failure. JACC Hear Fail 2018;6(4):329–39.

41. Valli G, Vizza CD, Onorati P, et al. Pathophysiological adaptations to walking and cycling in primary pulmonary hypertension. Eur J Appl Physiol 2008. https://doi.org/10.1007/s00421-007-0600-y.

42. Ma KA, Kahn SR, Akaberi A, et al. Serial imaging after pulmonary embolism and correlation with functional limitation at 12 months: Results of the ELOPE Study. Res Pract Thromb Haemost 2018;2(4):670–7.

43. Albaghdadi MS, Dudzinski DM, Giordano N, et al. Cardiopulmonary exercise testing in patients following massive and submassive pulmonary embolism. J Am Heart Assoc 2018;7(5):12–4.

44. Osman AF, Mehra MR, Lavie CJ, et al. The incremental prognostic importance of body fat adjusted peak oxygen consumption in chronic heart failure. J Am Coll Cardiol 2000;36(7):2126–31.

45. Yasunobu Y, Oudiz RJ, Sun XG, et al. End-tidal Pco2 abnormality and exercise limitation in patients with primary pulmonary hypertension. Chest 2005;127(5):1637–46.

46. Sun Xing-Guo, James E, Hansen RJO, et al. Exercise Pathophysiology in Patients With Primary Pulmonary Hypertension. Circulation 2001;104:429–35.

47. Dhakal BP, Malhotra R, Murphy RM, et al. Mechanisms of exercise intolerance in heart failure with preserved ejection fraction: The role of abnormal peripheral oxygen extraction. Circ Hear Fail 2015;8(2):286–94.

48. Jain CC, Borlaug BA. Performance and Interpretation of Invasive Hemodynamic Exercise Testing. Chest 2020;158(5):2119–29.

49. Lewis GD, Bossone E, Naeije R, et al. Pulmonary vascular hemodynamic response to exercise in cardiopulmonary diseases. Circulation 2013;128(13):1470–9.

50. Raza F, Kozitza C, Lechuga C, et al. Multimodality deep phenotyping methods to assess mechanisms of poor right ventricular-pulmonary artery coupling. Function 2022;3(4):zqac022.

51. Raza F, Dharmavaram N, Hess T, et al. Distinguishing exercise intolerance in early-stage pulmonary

hypertension with invasive exercise hemodynamics: Rest V E/V CO 2 and ETCO 2 identify pulmonary vascular disease. Clin Cardiol 2022;45(7): 742–51.

52. Kozitza CJ, Tao R. Pulmonary vascular distensibility with passive leg raise is comparable to exercise and predictive of clinical outcomes in pulmonary hypertension. Pulm Circ 2022;12(1): e12029.

53. Kovacs G, Herve P, Barbera JA, et al. An official European Respiratory Society statement: pulmonary haemodynamics during exercise. Eur Respir J 2017;50(5). https://doi.org/10.1183/13993003. 00578-2017.

54. Eisman AS, Shah RV, Dhakal BP, et al. Pulmonary Capillary Wedge Pressure Patterns During Exercise Predict Exercise Capacity and Incident Heart Failure. Circ Heart Fail 2018;11(5):e004750.

55. Enright PL. The Six-Minute Walk Test Introduction Standards and Indications 6-Minute Walk Test Versus Shuttle Walk Test Safety Variables Measured Conducting the Test Ensuring Quality Factors That Influence 6-Minute Walk Distance Interpreting the Results Improving the. Respir Care 2003;48(8):783–5. Available at: http://rc.rcjournal.com/content/respcare/48/8/783.full.pdf.

56. Holland AE, Spruit MA, Troosters T, et al. An official European respiratory society/American thoracic society technical standard: Field walking tests in chronic respiratory disease. Eur Respir J 2014;44(6):1428–46.

57. Singh SJ, Puhan MA, Andrianopoulos V, et al. An official systematic review of the European Respiratory Society/American Thoracic Society: Measurement properties of field walking tests in chronic respiratory disease. Eur Respir J 2014;44(6):1447–78.

58. Miyamoto S, Nagaya N, Satoh T, et al. Clinical correlates and prognostic significance of six-minute walk test in patients with primary pulmonary hypertension: Comparison with cardiopulmonary exercise testing. Am J Respir Crit Care Med 2000; 161(2 I):487–92.

59. Albaghdadi MS, Dudzinski DM, Giordano N, et al. Cardiopulmonary Exercise Testing in Patients Following Massive and Submassive Pulmonary Embolism. J Am Hear Assoc 2018;7(5). https://doi.org/10.1161/JAHA.117.006841.

60. Konstantinides SV, Vicaut E, Danays T, et al. Impact of Thrombolytic Therapy on the Long-Term Outcome of Intermediate-Risk Pulmonary Embolism. J Am Coll Cardiol 2017;69(12):1536–44.

61. Lewis AE, Gerstein NS, Venkataramani R. Evolving management trends and outcomes in catheter management of acute pulmonary embolism. J Cardiothorac Vasc Anesth 2022;36(8 Pt B): 3344–56.

62. Piazza G, Hohlfelder B, Harm PD, et al. A prospective, single-arm, multicenter trial of ultrasound-facilitated, catheter-directed, low-dose fibrinolysis for acute massive and submassive pulmonary embolism: the SEATTLE II study. JACC Cardiovasc Interv 2015;8(10):1382–92.

63. Kuo WT, Banerjee A, Kim PS, et al. Pulmonary embolism response to fragmentation, embolectomy, and catheter thrombolysis (PERFECT): Initial results from a prospective multicenter registry. Chest 2015;148(3):667–73.

64. Kucher N, Boekstegers P, Müller OJ, et al. Randomized, controlled trial of ultrasound-assisted catheter-directed thrombolysis for acute intermediate-risk pulmonary embolism. Circulation 2014;129(4):479–86.

65. Sahni S, Capozzi B, Iftikhar A, et al. Pulmonary rehabilitation and exercise in pulmonary arterial hypertension: An underutilized intervention. J Exerc Rehabil 2015;11(2):74–9.

66. Pandey A, Parashar A, Kumbhani D, et al. Exercise training in patients with heart failure and preserved ejection fraction: meta-analysis of randomized control trials. Circ Hear Fail 2015;8(1):33–40.

67. Group CW. Pulmonary rehabilitation for patients with chronic pulmonary disease (COPD): An evidence-based analysis. Ont Health Technol Assess Ser 2012;12(6):1–75.

68. Rehn TA, Munkvik M, Lunde PK, et al. Intrinsic skeletal muscle alterations in chronic heart failure patients: a disease-specific myopathy or a result of deconditioning? Hear Fail Rev 2012;17(3):421–36.

69. Löwe B, Gräfe K, Ufer C, et al. Anxiety and depression in patients with pulmonary hypertension. Psychosom Med 2004;66(6):831–6.

70. Haukeland-Parker S, Jervan O, Johannessen HH, et al. Pulmonary rehabilitation to improve physical capacity, dyspnea, and quality of life following pulmonary embolism (the PeRehab study): study protocol for a two-center randomized controlled trial. Trials 2021;22(1):1–9.

71. Gleditsch J, Jervan, Haukeland-Parker S, et al. Effects of pulmonary rehabilitation on cardiac magnetic resonance parameters in patients with persistent dyspnea following pulmonary embolism. IJC Hear Vasc 2022;40(March):100995.

72. Rolving N, Brocki BC, Bloch-Nielsen JR, et al. Effect of a physiotherapist-guided home-based exercise intervention on physical capacity and patient-reported outcomes among patients with acute pulmonary embolism: a randomized clinical trial. JAMA Netw Open 2020;3(2):e200064.

73. Nopp S, Klok FA, Moik F, et al. Outpatient pulmonary rehabilitation in patients with persisting symptoms after pulmonary embolism. J Clin Med 2020;9(6):1–12.

74. Fox BD, Kassirer M, Weiss I, et al. Ambulatory rehabilitation improves exercise capacity in patients with pulmonary hypertension. J Card Fail 2011;17(3):196–200.

75. O'Connor CM, Whellan DJ, Lee KL, et al. Efficacy and safety of exercise training in patients with chronic heart failure: HF-ACTION randomized controlled trial. JAMA 2009;301(14):1439–50.

76. Conraads VM, Pattyn N, De Maeyer C, et al. Aerobic interval training and continuous training equally improve aerobic exercise capacity in patients with coronary artery disease: The SAINTEX-CAD study. Int J Cardiol 2015;179:203–10.

77. Maddison R, Rawstorn JC, Stewart RAH, et al. Effects and costs of real-time cardiac telerehabilitation: Randomised controlled non-inferiority trial. Heart 2019;105(2):122–9.

78. Prabhakaran D, Chandrasekaran AM, Singh K, et al. Yoga-based cardiac rehabilitation after acute myocardial infarction: a randomized trial. J Am Coll Cardiol 2020;75(13):1551–61.

79. Ries AL, Make BJ, Lee SM, et al. The effects of pulmonary rehabilitation in the national emphysema treatment trial. Chest 2005;128(6):3799–809.

80. Cires-Drouet RS, Mayorga-Carlin M, Toursavadkohi S, et al. Safety of exercise therapy after acute pulmonary embolism. Phlebology 2020;35(10):824–32.

81. Dalal HM, Taylor RS, Jolly K, et al. The effects and costs of home-based rehabilitation for heart failure with reduced ejection fraction: the reach-hf multicentre randomized controlled trial. Eur J Prev Cardiol 2019;26(3):262–72.

82. Hillegass E, Puthoff M, Frese EM, et al. Role of physical therapists in the management of individuals at risk for or diagnosed with venous thromboembolism: Evidence-based clinical practice guideline. Phys Ther 2016;96(2):143–66.

83. Thompson PD. Exercise prescription and proscription for patients with coronary artery disease. Circulation 2005;112(15):2354–63.

84. Wenger NK. Current status of cardiac rehabilitation. J Am Coll Cardiol 2008;51(17):1619–31.

85. Cardiac rehabilitation programs. A statement for healthcare professionals from the American Heart Association. Circulation 1994;90(3):1602–10.

86. Saltin B, Blomqvist G, Mitchell JH, et al. Response to exercise after bed rest and after training. Circulation 1968;38(5 Suppl):VII1–78. Available at: https://www.ncbi.nlm.nih.gov/pubmed/5696236.

87. Naughton J, Lategola MT, Shanbour K. A physical rehabilitation program for cardiac patients: a progress report. Am J Med Sci 1966;252(5):545–53. Available at: https://www.ncbi.nlm.nih.gov/pubmed/5924755.

88. Bethell HJ. Cardiac rehabilitation: from Hellerstein to the millennium. Int J Clin Pract 2000;54(2):92–7.

Available at: https://www.ncbi.nlm.nih.gov/pubmed/10824363.

89. Anderson L, Oldridge N, Thompson DR, et al. Exercise-Based Cardiac Rehabilitation for Coronary Heart Disease: Cochrane Systematic Review and Meta-Analysis. J Am Coll Cardiol 2016;67(1):1–12.

90. Mezzani A, Hamm LF, Jones AM, et al. Aerobic exercise intensity assessment and prescription in cardiac rehabilitation: a joint position statement of the European Association for Cardiovascular Prevention and Rehabilitation, the American Association of Cardiovascular and Pulmonary Rehabilitat. Eur J Prev Cardiol 2013;20(3):442–67.

91. Wisloff U, Stoylen A, Loennechen JP, et al. Superior cardiovascular effect of aerobic interval training versus moderate continuous training in heart failure patients: a randomized study. Circulation 2007;115(24):3086–94.

92. Moholdt T, Aamot IL, Granoien I, et al. Aerobic interval training increases peak oxygen uptake more than usual care exercise training in myocardial infarction patients: a randomized controlled study. Clin Rehabil 2012;26(1):33–44.

93. Taylor JL, Holland DJ, Keating SE, et al. Short-term and Long-term Feasibility, Safety, and Efficacy of High-Intensity Interval Training in Cardiac Rehabilitation: The FITR Heart Study Randomized Clinical Trial. JAMA Cardiol 2020;5(12):1382–9.

94. Guazzi M, Reina G, Tumminello G, et al. Improvement of alveolar-capillary membrane diffusing capacity with exercise training in chronic heart failure. J Appl Physiol 2004;97(5):1866–73.

95. Andrade DC, Arce-Alvarez A, Parada F, et al. Acute effects of high-intensity interval training session and endurance exercise on pulmonary function and cardiorespiratory coupling. Physiol Rep 2020;8(15):e14455.

96. Tasoulis A, Papazachou O, Dimopoulos S, et al. Effects of interval exercise training on respiratory drive in patients with chronic heart failure. Respir Med 2010;104(10):1557–65.

97. Thijssen DH, Dawson EA, Black MA, et al. Brachial artery blood flow responses to different modalities of lower limb exercise. Med Sci Sport Exerc 2009;41(5):1072–9.

98. Calverley TA, Ogoh S, Marley CJ, et al. HIITing the brain with exercise: mechanisms, consequences and practical recommendations. J Physiol 2020;598(13):2513–30.

99. Barnes JN, Schmidt JE, Nicholson WT, et al. Cyclooxygenase inhibition abolishes age-related differences in cerebral vasodilator responses to hypercapnia. J Appl Physiol 2012;112(11):1884–90.

100. Green DJ, Hopman MT, Padilla J, et al. Vascular Adaptation to Exercise in Humans: Role of Hemodynamic Stimuli. Physiol Rev 2017;97(2):495–528.

101. Del Buono MG, Arena R, Borlaug BA, et al. Exercise Intolerance in Patients With Heart Failure: JACC State-of-the-Art Review. J Am Coll Cardiol 2019;73(17):2209–25.

102. Lundby C, Montero D, Joyner M. Biology of VO2 max: looking under the physiology lamp. Acta Physiol 2017;220(2):218–28.

103. Haykowsky MJ, Brubaker PH, Stewart KP, et al. Effect of endurance training on the determinants of peak exercise oxygen consumption in elderly patients with stable compensated heart failure and preserved ejection fraction. J Am Coll Cardiol 2012;60(2):120–8.

104. Levinger I, Bronks R, Cody DV, et al. The effect of resistance training on left ventricular function and structure of patients with chronic heart failure. Int J Cardiol 2005;105(2):159–63.

105. Palevo G, Keteyian SJ, Kang M, et al. Resistance exercise training improves heart function and physical fitness in stable patients with heart failure. J Cardiopulm Rehabil Prev 2009;29(5):294–8.

106. Ozaki H, Loenneke J, Thiebaud R, et al. Resistance training induced increase in VO2max in young and older subjects. Eur Rev Aging Phys Act 2013;10. https://doi.org/10.1007/s11556-013-0120-1.

107. Liu T, Chan AW, Liu YH, et al. Effects of Tai Chi-based cardiac rehabilitation on aerobic endurance, psychosocial well-being, and cardiovascular risk reduction among patients with coronary heart disease: A systematic review and meta-analysis. Eur J Cardiovasc Nurs 2018;17(4):368–83.

108. Borg GA V. Physical Performance and Perceived Exertion. Lund; Copenhagen: Berlingska boktryckeriet, C.W.K. Gleerup ; E. Munksgaard; 1962.

109. Konstantinides SV, Meyer G, Bueno H, et al. 2019 ESC Guidelines for the diagnosis and management of acute pulmonary embolism developed in collaboration with the European respiratory society (ERS). Eur Heart J 2020;41(4):543–603.

110. Ramirez-Jimenez M, Fernandez-Elias V, Morales-Palomo F, et al. Intense aerobic exercise lowers blood pressure in individuals with metabolic syndrome taking antihypertensive medicine. Blood Press Monit 2018;23(5):230–6.

111. Ramirez-Jimenez M, Morales-Palomo F, Ortega JF, et al. Effects of intense aerobic exercise and/or antihypertensive medication in individuals with metabolic syndrome. Scand J Med Sci Sport 2018;28(9):2042–51.

112. Maddison R, Rawstorn JC, Rolleston A, et al. The remote exercise monitoring trial for exercise-based cardiac rehabilitation (REMOTE-CR): A randomised controlled trial protocol. BMC Publ Health 2014;14(1):1–8.

113. Anderson L, Sharp GA, Norton RJ, et al. Home-based versus centre-based cardiac rehabilitation. Cochrane Database Syst Rev 2017;6:CD007130.

114. Bayoumy K, Gaber M, Elshafeey A, et al. Smart wearable devices in cardiovascular care: where we are and how to move forward. Nat Rev Cardiol 2021;18(8):581–99.

Technical Considerations for Performing Safe and Effective Balloon Pulmonary Angioplasty in Patients with Chronic Thromboembolic Pulmonary Hypertension

Kazuya Hosokawa, MD, PhD[a],*, Yuzo Yamasaki, MD, PhD[b], Kohtaro Abe, MD, PhD[a]

KEYWORDS

- Chronic thromboembolic pulmonary hypertension • Balloon pulmonary angioplasty
- Pulmonary thromboembolism

KEY POINTS

- Five-year survival rate of chronic thromboembolic pulmonary hypertension (CTEPH) with anticoagulation alone is less than 50% in patients with mean pulmonary artery pressure (PAP) above 30 mm Hg.
- Forty percent of patients with CTEPH are not candidates for the first-line treatment of pulmonary endarterectomy, because of distal lesions or age.
- Balloon pulmonary angioplasty, a catheter-based intervention, is increasingly being used worldwide for the treatment of inoperable CTEPH.
- Strategy of balloon pulmonary angioplasty has evolved, which ensured safety (procedure-related mortality <1%). Staged balloon pulmonary angioplasty using different balloon sizes for mean baseline PAP ≥35 mm Hg and <35 mm Hg is crucial.
- Five-year survival rate of balloon pulmonary angioplasty for inoperable CTEPH has improved to 90%, which is comparable to that of operable CTEPH.

INTRODUCTION

Chronic thromboembolic pulmonary hypertension (CTEPH) is classified as group 4 pulmonary hypertension.[1–3] In CTEPH, stenoses or occlusions of the pulmonary arteries owing to organized thrombi can cause elevations in pulmonary artery resistance and pressure, resulting in pulmonary hypertension. Previously, CTEPH patients with mean pulmonary arterial pressure (PAP) higher than 30 mm Hg had extremely poor prognosis, with survival of only

10% if left untreated.[4] Pulmonary endarterectomy is the first-line therapy; however, patients deemed un1suitable for pulmonary endarterectomy owing to lesion inaccessibility, aging, or comorbidities had poor prognosis and limited treatment options.[1] Based on the 2007 to 2009 data of an international registry, 63% of the patients with CTEPH were considered operable and 36% were considered inoperable, with 57% undergoing surgery.[5] In 2001, a small clinical trial of balloon pulmonary angioplasty (BPA) was first reported as a treatment

---

[a] Faculty of Cardiovascular Medicine, Graduate School of Medical Sciences, Kyushu University, 3-1-1 Maidashi, Higashi-Ku, Fukuoka 812-8582, Japan; [b] Department of Clinical Radiology, Graduate School of Medical Sciences, Kyushu University, 3-1-1 Maidashi, Higashi-Ku, Fukuoka 812-8582, Japan
* Corresponding author:
E-mail address: hosokawa.kazuya.712@m.kyushu-u.ac.jp

Intervent Cardiol Clin 12 (2023) 367–380
https://doi.org/10.1016/j.iccl.2023.02.003
2211-7458/23/© 2023 Elsevier Inc. All rights reserved.

in 18 patients with inoperable CTEPH.[6] Despite improvements in pulmonary hypertension and functional performance, that study reported high complication rates, including lung injury (61.1%), need of mechanical ventilatory support (16.7%), and 1 procedure-related mortality. Because the complications were considered disproportionate to the potential benefits, BPA was initially not widely accepted. In 2012, Mizoguchi and colleagues[7] reported refinement of BPA techniques. Subsequently, several studies have demonstrated that BPA improved exercise tolerance, hemodynamics, and eventually survival (2-year survival, 85%–100%), with lower perioperative mortality (0%–3.4%).[8] Based on these clinical observations, the European Respiratory Society statement on CTEPH management recommended BPA as a therapeutic option for inoperable patients with CTEPH.[3] Thus, the BPA procedure has been developed worldwide. In this review, the authors highlight the technical considerations for conducting safe and effective BPA to avoid BPA-related complications in patients with inoperable CTEPH.

DISCUSSION
General Treatment Strategy for Chronic Thromboembolic Pulmonary Hypertension and Indications of Balloon Pulmonary Angioplasty

The current treatment algorithm for CTEPH is shown in Fig. 1.[1] CTEPH is diagnosed in patients with mean PAP of 25 mm Hg or higher despite appropriate conventional oral anticoagulation therapy with vitamin K antagonists for at least 3 months from the time of the first observation of pulmonary thrombi. The algorithm recommends multidisciplinary assessment of operability in a pulmonary hypertension referral center by a team consisting of a surgeon experienced in pulmonary endarterectomy, a pulmonary hypertension specialist, a BPA interventionist, and CTEPH-trained radiologists. The most distinct difference between pulmonary endarterectomy and BPA is the perception of indication based on lesions. In pulmonary endarterectomy, the organized thrombi are considered as a whole, and the indication for surgery is determined by the extent and location of the thrombi. On the other hand, the indication for BPA is considered for each individual artery according to the type, distribution, and location of the lesion. As shown in Fig. 1, patients with operable CTEPH should receive pulmonary endarterectomy as the first-line treatment. For those deemed inoperable, the best level of evidence supports initiation of medical therapy or consideration of BPA. Patients with persistent or recurrent symptomatic pulmonary hypertension after pulmonary endarterectomy should receive medical therapy and be considered for BPA or repeat endarterectomy in cases of significant reocclusion. Based on the evidence obtained from prospective clinical trials, pulmonary arterial hypertension-specific drugs have been approved for pulmonary hypertension without or after pulmonary endarterectomy or BPA in inoperable patients with CTEPH.[9–11] However, the efficacy and safety of these drugs for preventing BPA-related complications in patients who are scheduled to undergo BPA procedure have not been established. An ongoing international BPA registry will provide more detailed long-term information on the use of medications for pulmonary hypertension before and after BPA (NCT03245268).

The Japanese Circulation Society statement regarding BPA describes the criteria for BPA candidates as follows: (1) Cases unsuitable for pulmonary endarterectomy (surgically inaccessible lesions, surgically accessible but inoperable because of comorbidities, and residual or recurrent pulmonary hypertension after pulmonary endarterectomy); (2) inadequate response to conventional therapy (World Health Organization functional class III or higher after conventional therapy, mean PAP $\geq$30 mm Hg, or pulmonary vascular resistance [PVR] $\geq$ 300 dyne*s*cm^{-5}); (3) patients who provide informed consent (patients who select BPA after fully understanding the risks and benefits of both BPA and pulmonary endarterectomy); and (4) cases without serious complications, multiorgan failure, or iodine allergy.[12] Recently, several studies have demonstrated that BPA also improved exercise tolerance as well as exercise-induced pulmonary hypertension with increased slope of the pulmonary arterial pressure–flow relationship in patients with chronic thromboembolic disease, who have similar symptoms and perfusion defects as CTEPH but without pulmonary hypertension at rest.[13–15] Chronic thromboembolic disease and CTEPH presumably represent a disease spectrum with the same pathophysiologic mechanism. However, the natural history of chronic thromboembolic disease is unknown, and there is no evidence that chronic thromboembolic disease evolves to CTEPH. Therefore, the current international statement has not yet recommended BPA as a treatment for symptomatic chronic thromboembolic disease.[3]

History of Balloon Pulmonary Angioplasty
The milestones in the history of BPA include the first case of BPA for CTEPH reported by

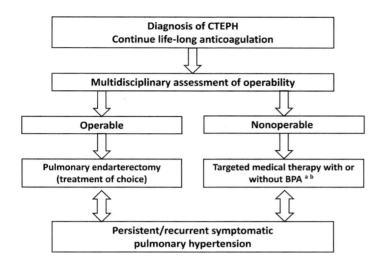

Fig. 1. Treatment algorithm for CTEPH modified from Ref.[1] [a]Treatment assessment may differ depending on the level of expertise. [b]BPA without medical therapy can be considered in selected cases.

Voorburg and colleagues[16] in 1988, who dilated 4 lesions in a 30-year-old patient, reducing mean PAP and PVR (from 46 to 35 mm Hg and from 688 to 532 dyne*s*cm^{-5}, respectively). This report provided the proof of concept for BPA. Thirteen years after the first case report, Feinstein and colleagues[6] summarized the first case series of 18 inoperable patients with CTEPH, in whom they dilated an average of 6 (range 1–12) lesions in 2.6 (range 1–5) sessions per patient. This series established the efficacy of the procedure; the New York Heart Association class improved from 3.3 to 1.8 (P<.001), 6-minute walk distance increased from 209 to 497 yards (P<.0001), and mean PAP decreased from 43.0 ± 12.1 to 33.7 ± 10.2 mm Hg (P = .007). However, 11 (61.1%) patients developed reperfusion pulmonary edema, including 3 (16.7%) who required mechanical ventilation and 1 (5.6%) death. These results conclude the need to improve the safety of this procedure, because the risk-benefit balance of BPA is unacceptable compared with that of pulmonary endarterectomy with mortality reported to be as low as 2.2%. In 2012, Mizoguchi and colleagues[7] refined the strategy specially to address safety in 68 inoperable patients with CTEPH. They refined 2 points: (1) Using intravascular ultrasound to obtain accurate target vessel diameters, (2) limiting treatment area per session to avoid fatal pulmonary reperfusion injury but repeating multiple sessions to cover all the lesions. Their strategy required an average of 4 (2–8) sessions per patient, and an average of 3 (1–14) vessels were dilated per session. The World Health Organization functional class

improved from 3 to 2 (P<.01), and mean PAP decreased from 45.4 ± 9.6 to 24.0 ± 6.4 mm Hg (P<.01). Forty-one patients (60%) developed reperfusion pulmonary injury after BPA, but mechanical ventilation was required in only 4 patients. The mortality was 1.5%. Since this report, BPA as a treatment option for inoperable CTEPH has been used worldwide. CTEPH centers around the world have reported the results of BPA for inoperable CTEPH. Although some regional differences are observed, similar efficacy and safety are confirmed (Table 1).[17–21] The BPA strategy at the time of Mizoguchi's report was to limit the area of BPA and repeat the procedure to avoid extensive pulmonary edema even if reperfusion pulmonary edema occurred, acknowledging a high probability of the occurrence of reperfusion pulmonary edema. Thereafter, BPA strategies have evolved further. In 2013, Inami and colleagues[22] reported that baseline PVR and flow grade improvement before and after balloon dilation were closely related to the incidence of reperfusion pulmonary edema. In addition, they reported that pressure-guided BPA would help to avoid reperfusion pulmonary edema. They also found that reperfusion pulmonary edema did not occur at peripheral pressure of 33 mm Hg or lower immediately after BPA.[23] Based on these 2 studies, the current BPA strategy in patients with mean PAP of 35 mm Hg or above before BPA is to dilate as many lesions as possible with an undersized balloon leaving a pressure gradient to avoid excessive blood flow increase to the peripheral pulmonary artery.[24] When the mean PAP drops to below 35 mm Hg, staged BPA sessions can

Table 1
Balloon pulmonary angioplasty outcomes from various countries

First Author Publication, Year	Location	Patients, n	BPA Sessions, n	Mean or Median Age, y	FC Improvement, % of I or II	6MWD Improvement, m	Reduction in Mean PAP, mm Hg	Lung Injury, % MV/ECMO, %	Mortality Rate <30 d After BPA, %
Ogawa et al,[17] 2017	Japan	308	1408	61.5 ± 12.5	19.2% → 85.6%	318 ± 122 → 401 ± 105	43.2 ± 11.0 → 24.3 ± 6.4	17.8 5.5/2.9	2.6
Olsson et al,[18] 2017	Germany	56	266	65 (range, 55–74)	15% → 73%	358 ± 108 → 391 ± 108	40 ± 12 → 33 ± 11	0.8 Not reported	1.8
Brenot et al,[19] 2019	France	184	1006	63 ± 14	35.3% → 78.7%	396 ± 120 → 441 ± 104	43.9 ± 9.5 → 31.6 ± 9.0	9.1 0.4/0.3	2.2
Hoole et al,[21] 2020	United Kingdom	30	3 (IQR 1–6) sessions/patients	63.5 ± 11.6	20% → 100%	366 ± 107 → 440 ± 94	44.7 ± 11.0 → 34.4 ± 8.3	10.5 0/0	0
Cale et al,[20] 2021	Portugal	11	57	66 ± 12	77.8% → 100%	420 ± 51 → 462 ± 55	34.8 ± 12.5 → 26.0 ± 6.4	5.3 0/0	0

Abbreviations: 6MWD, 6-minute walk distance; ECMO, extracorporeal membrane oxygenation; FC, functional class; IQR, interquartile range; MV, mechanical ventilation.

be done using larger balloons to dilate lesions. This staged BPA procedure has been established as a safe and efficient BPA strategy that does not cause reperfusion pulmonary edema.[25]

Anatomy and Normal Variant of Pulmonary Artery

Understanding the pulmonary artery tree and normal variations is crucial to perform a safe and effective BPA. The main pulmonary artery arises from the pulmonary valve attached to the right ventricle and runs craniodorsally, bifurcating into the right and left pulmonary arteries below the carina of trachea. The right pulmonary artery turns right almost horizontally, and the left pulmonary artery courses craniodorsally passing over the left main bronchus; therefore, the left hilum is higher than the right hilum. Each pulmonary artery divides into lobar branches and subsequently into segmental and subsegmental branches. Segmental and subsegmental pulmonary arteries are named based on the bronchopulmonary segments that they feed. Numerous variations of pulmonary arterial branching exist. Variations are more common in pulmonary branches in the upper lobes than those in the lower lobes.[26,27]

Right pulmonary artery

The right upper lobe is supplied by the truncus superior and ascending arteries arising from the interlobar artery. The first branch of right pulmonary artery is always the truncus superior that feeds the right upper lobe, including the apical segment (S1). Apart from the truncus superior, ascending arteries also supply the right upper lobe in most cases[26–28] (Fig. 2A, B). The truncus superior rarely feeds the whole right upper lobe (10%).[28] Occasionally, there may be segmental supply to the upper lobe from the middle lobe artery or A6.

The middle lobe segmental arteries arise from the right interlobar artery. Both separate (53.4%) and common origins (42.5%) of the arteries to the lateral (S4) and medial (S5) segments of the middle lobe are observed.[29] For separate origins, A4a or A4 occasionally originates after branching A6. Subsequently, after the branch to the superior segment (S6) separates posteriorly, the common basal trunk (basal pulmonary artery) ultimately divides into 4 terminal branches that supply the medial basal (S7), anterior basal (S8), lateral basal (S9), and posterior basal segments (S10). Occasionally, there may be 2 or 3 separate branches to the superior segment (S6) (20%).[29]

Left pulmonary artery

Segmental branches typically arise from the left pulmonary artery without forming a trunk; therefore, there are more anatomic variations on the left than on the right. The first branch of left pulmonary artery is normally the branch to the anterior segment (S3). The artery to the apicoposterior segment (S1+2) has 4 variations (A1+2abc; A1+2a+b and A1+2c; A1+2a and A1+2b+c; A1+2a, A1+2b, and A1+2c), and some of them occasionally form a common trunk with A3.[30]

Typically, lingula is supplied by 1 or 2 branches of the left pulmonary artery. The origin of the lingular artery has 2 important variations. First, the mediastinal lingular artery arises from near the origin of A3 as the first or second branch of left pulmonary artery (Fig. 2C). Second, the interlobar pulmonary artery arises from the interlobar aspect of the left pulmonary artery after branching A1+2 and A3 (Fig. 2D); occasionally it originates after branching A6 or A8 (30%).[31] The interlobar type is most common (72.5%), followed by both interlobar and mediastinal type (17.5%), and mediastinal type (10%).[29]

After the branch to the superior segment (S6) separates posteriorly, the common basal trunk ultimately divides into 3 terminal branches that supply the anterior basal (S8), lateral basal (S9), and posterior basal segments (S10). S7 and A7 do not exist in the left lung. Similar to the right side, there are sometimes 2 or 3 separate branches to the superior segment (S6). Mediastinal basal pulmonary artery is rare but an important variation that arises from the origin of A3 (and mediastinal lingular artery) and supplies the basal segments. This variation may occur as a replacement (mediastinal basal artery without original basal artery) or duplication (mediastinal basal artery with the original basal artery) (Fig. 2E, F).

Physiologic Basis for Evaluating Balloon Pulmonary Angioplasty

The goal of BPA is to improve prognosis and exercise tolerance. As with pulmonary endarterectomy, there are no randomized controlled trials that evaluate whether BPA is effective in improving prognosis and exercise capacity. However, a multicenter retrospective study from Japanese centers specialized in BPA reported the outcome of BPA in patients with inoperable CTEPH as follows: mean PAP improved from 43.2 ± 11.0 mm Hg at baseline to 24.3 ± 6.4 mm Hg at follow-up 425.5 ± 280.9 days after BPA, and 3-year

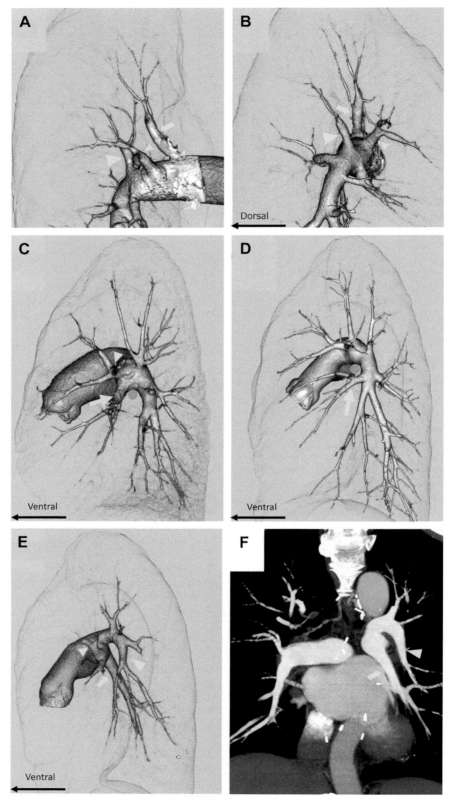

Fig. 2. Normal variants of pulmonary artery. (*A, B*) Coronal (*A*) and sagittal (*B*) images of 3D volume rendering of right pulmonary artery in CT pulmonary angiography showing the 3 branches of right pulmonary artery supplying the right upper lobe. Arrows indicate truncus superior supplying the apical segment (S1). Large arrowheads indicate ascending artery supplying the posterior segment (S2). Small arrowheads indicate another ascending artery

survival rate was 94.5% (95% CI, 89.3%–97.3%).[17] The natural history of patients with CTEPH on anticoagulation alone was reported by Riedel and colleagues[32] in 1982. Patients with mean PAP above 30 mm Hg had a 3-year survival rate of less than 70% and a 5-year survival rate of less than 50%. A prospective European registry reported by Delcroix and colleagues[33] in 2016, which was conducted before BPA was widely used, also reported a 3-year survival rate of 70% (95% CI, 64–76) in patients with CTEPH who did not undergo surgery. Therefore, it is plausible to consider that BPA treatment strategies have improved the prognosis of inoperable CTEPH. As shown in the BPA results from Japan, France, Germany, United Kingdom, and Portugal (see **Table 1**), improvements in functional class and 6-minute walk distance were observed in all regions, as well as favorable early low mortalities. Mean PAP and PVR, which are surrogate markers for prognosis and exercise tolerance, respectively, can be measured easily to assess the acute effects of BPA. Particularly, mean PAP below 30 mm Hg is commonly recognized as a mandatory goal of BPA, because mean PAP above 30 mm Hg was associated with long-term poor prognosis in the epidemiologic study reported by Riedel and colleagues.[32] On the other hand, in a series of 18 patients with chronic thromboembolic disease but no pulmonary hypertension at rest (mean PAP below 25 mm Hg) who had median age of 58 years (interquartile range 44–68 years), BPA improved 6-minute walk distance significantly (from 408 [interquartile range 358–468] m to 444 [interquartile range 380–566] m, $P = .03$), suggesting room for improvement of exercise tolerance in middle-aged patients.[15] The goals of BPA in middle-aged patients with CTEPH might be to normalize PAP at rest (mean PAP below 25 mm Hg, ideally below 20 mm Hg) and to increase reserve pulmonary vascular bed.

Measuring mean PAP and PVR, which are significant indices of prognosis and exercise tolerance, respectively, before and after BPA is routinely performed to evaluate the acute effect of BPA. However, this concept has 2 pitfalls.

First, BPA mainly lowers mean PAP and PVR in patients with severe CTEPH compared with those with mild CTEPH. When PVR is broken down into 20 vascular resistances (R1 to R20), one for each segmental branch, the pulmonary circulation can be considered as a parallel circuit. Then, PVR is represented by R_n as follows:

$$PVR = \frac{1}{\frac{1}{R1} + \frac{1}{R2} + \cdots \frac{1}{R20}}$$

To simplify the calculation, it is assumed that all vascular resistances are equal ($R1 = R2 = \cdots = R20 = R_{seg}$). Because the vascular resistance R_n of the obstructed branch increases significantly and $1/R_n$ can be assumed to be 0, then, the following equation holds:

$$PVR = \frac{R_{seg}}{\text{Number of patent segmental arteries}}$$

Given $R_{seg} = 40.0$ WU, the PVR for a person with 20 patent segmental arteries is PVR 2.0 WU, which is the normal value of PVR.

$$PVR = \frac{40}{\text{Number of open segmental arteries}}$$

Simplifying the above equation, the relationship between PVR and the number of patent segmental arteries is a hyperbola, as shown in **Fig. 3**. Because mean PAP is PVR multiplied by the resting cardiac output (≈ 5.0 L/min) plus pulmonary artery wedge pressure (≈ 5 mm Hg), within the compensated range of the right ventricle, the relationship between mean PAP and number of patent segmental arteries is a hyperbolic curve, as for PVR (see **Fig. 3**).

When comparing the impact of a BPA procedure (revascularization of 2 segmental arteries) between severe CTEPH with only 4 patent segmental arteries and mild CTEPH with 10 patent segmental arteries, the decreases in PVR and mean PAP are markedly greater in severe CTEPH than in mild CTEPH (see **Fig. 3**). This framework would explain why later BPA sessions reduce PVR and mean PAP less than earlier sessions. The second pitfall is that PVR and mean PAP sometimes do not improve immediately after a successful BPA. Although the detailed

---

supplying the anterior segment (S3). (*C, D*) Sagittal images of 3D volume rendering of left pulmonary artery in CT pulmonary angiography. (*C*) Mediastinal lingular artery (*arrow*) arising next to A3 (*arrowhead*). (*D*) Interlobar lingular artery (*arrow*) arising from left interlobar pulmonary artery. Note the relationship of each lingular artery and left upper lobe bronchus (*blue circle*). (*E, F*) Sagittal image of 3D volume rendering of left pulmonary artery (*E*) and coronal image of maximum intensity projection (*F*) in CT pulmonary angiography showing left original basal pulmonary artery (A8i, A9i, A10i) (*large arrowheads*) and (duplicated) mediastinal basal pulmonary artery (A8ii, A9ii, A10ii) (*arrows*) that arise from the origin of A3 (*small arrowhead*) with mediastinal lingular artery.

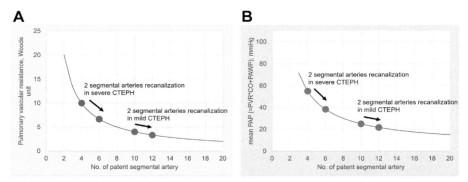

Fig. 3. Relationship of PVR and mean PAP with the number of patent segmental arteries. (A) Relationship between PVR and number of patent segmental arteries. (B) Relationship between mean PAP and number of patent segmental arteries. Both relationships are theoretically hyperbolic when the pulmonary circulation is represented as a simple parallel circuit consisting of 20 segmental branches. The impact of BPA (revascularization of 2 segmental arteries) is compared between severe CTEPH with only 4 patient segmental arteries and mild CTEPH with 10 patent segmental arteries. Decreases in PVR and mean PAP in severe CTEPH are markedly greater that the decreases in mild CTEPH. CO, cardiac output; PAWP, pulmonary artery wedge pressure.

mechanisms are unclear, it has been suggested that shrinkage of the lesion vessels may be involved in chronic occlusive lesions or long-standing stenotic lesions. Spontaneous vessel dilation with delayed reduction in PAP and PVR after recanalization has been observed.[34,35]

Tools for Balloon Pulmonary Angioplasty

There are no dedicated devices for BPA. General devices for peripheral intervention are used. Generally, access is via internal jugular vein or femoral vein. The BPA system is characterized by a short outer sheath that is placed at the access site and a long inner sheath with the tip placed at the right and left pulmonary arteries (blue arrowheads in Fig. 4). Typical examples of guiding catheter, wire, and balloon catheters used in BPA are shown in Table 2. Because the long inner sheath must reach the left and right pulmonary arteries, the length must be selected according to height. Two types of guiding catheters are usually used: one is mildly curved, such as Judkins right catheter; and the other is curved at greater than 90°, such as Judkins left catheter (see Fig. 4). If the guiding catheter cannot reach the target vessel, the target vessel may be selected with a wire, and the devices may be advanced in the order of balloon catheter followed by guide extension catheter to engage with the guide extension catheter. Guide extension catheters are useful for deep engagement to allow selective pulmonary arteriography and to reduce the amount of contrast media. Wire selection is pivotal for safe BPA, because the stretching and shrinking of the pulmonary artery synchronous with respiration and the pulsatile movement of the guiding catheter owing to heartbeat are factors that can lead to wire perforation. Wire perforations are common even in modern BPA, with a rate of 2%.[17] The first line wires have a soft tip (tip load <1 g) and no hydrophilic coating. Ringlike stenosis and web are usually crossed using a first-line wire. If there is a microchannel for the tip to dive into, subtotal occlusions can be crossed with a tip load less than 3 g, using a balloon catheter support technique (Fig. 5). Total occlusion without a microchannel (pouch defect) requires perforation of the occlusion cap, which requires a tapered wire or wire with heavier tip load in addition to a microcatheter. Because of the low success rate and high complication rate of BPA for total occlusion lesions,[36] the need for BPA itself should be considered in terms of the risk-benefit balance. In balloon catheter selection, because BPA does not require high-pressure dilation as in coronary artery intervention, semicompliant balloon catheters that allow adjustment of balloon size according to the dilation pressure are commonly used. Because vascular stents are not used in CTEPH treatment, accurate vessel sizing by intravascular imaging devices is not mandatory. Simple angiography-guided balloon sizing and dilation pressure are conducted to save time and cost. Rather than intravascular imaging-guided exact balloon sizing, undersized dilation is critical to avoid reperfusion pulmonary edema in patients with mean PAP higher than 35 mm Hg. If time and cost allow, pressure-guided BPA using the Rapid Exchange FFR Micro-Catheter (Nuvvus II Rapid Exchange FFR MicroCatheter; ACIST Medical Systems Inc, Eden Prairie, MN) will ideally ensure safety (peripheral pressure ≤33 mm Hg) and efficacy (target ratio of distal pressure/proximal pressure >0.7–0.8).[22,23]

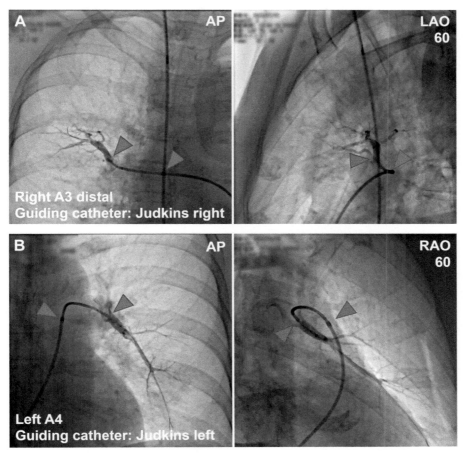

Fig. 4. Positioning of long inner sheaths and guiding catheters in right and left pulmonary artery. (A) BPA of right pulmonary arteries via jugular venous access using Judkins right catheter. (B) BPA of left pulmonary arteries via femoral venous access using Judkins left catheter. Red arrowhead indicates the tip of the guiding catheter. Blue arrowhead indicates the tip of the long inner sheath.

Treatment Strategy for Balloon Pulmonary Angioplasty

Improvements in surgical techniques in centers specialized in pulmonary endarterectomy have expanded the pool of patients who are candidates for pulmonary endarterectomy and improved the outcomes of pulmonary endarterectomy in patients with distal disease comparable to those in patients with proximal disease.[37] However, 40% of patients with CTEPH are considered inoperable. Furthermore, up to 51% of the patients will experience persistent/recurrent CTEPH after surgery.[5,38] Consequently, more than one-half of all patients with CTEPH are eligible for BPA. The latest BPA strategy is illustrated in Fig. 6. A candidate for BPA is first administered riociguat. The efficacy and safety of riociguat compared with BPA for inoperable CTEPH have been investigated in 2 randomized controlled trials: the 124-patient

RACE trial (NCT02634203) in France[39] and the MR BPA trial (UMIN000019549)[40] in Japan studying approximately 60 patients. The RACE trial was a crossover-controlled trial that investigated whether riociguat or BPA should be given first, and the interim report of the trial showed that although final PVR improved to the same degree regardless of the initial treatment, the group that initially received riociguat had less severe adverse events than the group that initially underwent BPA (initial riociguat 2.5% vs initial BPA 14%; $P = .0062$). BPA has been associated with bleeding complications, such as wire perforation, as well as reperfusion pulmonary edema. Preemptive treatment with riociguat is recommended to prepare for safe BPA by lowering the baseline PAP.

A good understanding of the pulmonary arterial anatomy of the patients is crucial to perform BPA efficiently. Selective pulmonary angiography

Table 2
Common balloon pulmonary angioplasty tools

Device	Size		Shape, Specifications, Purpose, and Other
Outer sheath	8F diameter, 10 cm long		Straight, placement for access site
Inner sheath	6F diameter, 70–90 cm long		Straight, placement for main right or left PA
Preshaped guiding catheters	6F diameter	Right A7 Left A1-5	Judkins left, and similar (largely curved shape)
		Others	Judkins right, and similar (mildly curved shape)
Wires	0.014 inch	1st line	Tip load <1 g without hydrophilic coating
		2nd line	Tip load 1–3 g with hydrophilic coating
Balloon catheters	Subsegmental artery	2.0–3.0 mm diameter	Semicompliant
	Segmental artery	4.0–6.0 mm diameter	Semicompliant
Optional tools	Guide extension catheter		For segmental pulmonary angiography
	Intravascular ultrasound imaging		For accurate measurement of vessel diameter
	Rapid-Exchange FFR Microcatheter[a]		For pressure-guided BPA
	Microcatheter		For totally occluded lesions

Abbreviations: FFR, fractional flow reserve; PA, pulmonary artery.
[a] ACIST Medical Systems Inc, Nuvvus II Rapid Exchange FFR microcatheter.

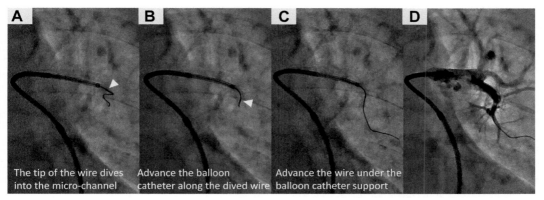

Fig. 5. Balloon catheter-assisted wiring. (*A*) Tip of the wire dives into a microchannel. (*B*) The balloon catheter is advanced up to the entrance of the microchannel. (*C*) The wire passes across the lesion under support of the balloon catheter. (*D*) Final segmental angiogram. Arrowhead indicates the tip of the balloon catheter.

should be performed on all segmental branches, as there are stenotic or occlusive lesions in more than 50% of the pulmonary vessels in CTEPH.[41] Major anatomic variants are commonly seen in right A3 and left A4 (see Fig. 2), which are often missed without anatomic imaging, such as 3-dimensional (3D) computed tomographic (CT) pulmonary angiography. As discussed in the previous

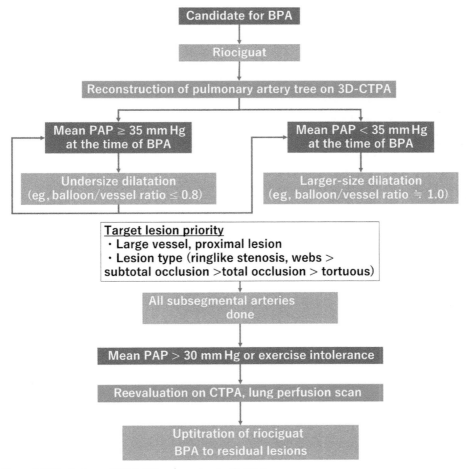

Fig. 6. Current BPA strategy. CTPA, CT pulmonary angiogram.

section, different balloon catheters should be selected for mean PAP of 35 mm Hg or above and for PAP below 35 mm Hg before BPA. Undersized dilatation is required when mean PAP is 35 mm Hg or above. If time and cost permit, pressure-guided BPA is helpful to ensure proper dilatation by monitoring peripheral pressure at 33 mm Hg or lower. In case of mean PAP below 35 mm Hg, larger dilation up to the size of the vessel diameter may be performed. Ringlike stenosis, web, and subtotal occlusion, which have lower complication rates and higher success rates, are candidate target lesions in early BPA sessions, compared with total occlusion or tortuous lesions (success rate and complication rate: ringlike stenosis, 100% and 1.6%; webs, 98.7% and 2.2%; subtotal occlusion, 86.5% and 15.5%; total occlusion, 52.2% and 6.0%; tortuous lesions, 63.6% and 43.2%, respectively).[36] Total occlusion or tortuous lesions should be performed after all the easier lesions have been treated and after considering the risk-benefit ratio if residual pulmonary hypertension is present or if exercise tolerance remains unsatisfactory. Some potential treatment strategies for total occlusion, such as CT pulmonary angiogram to identify the occluded peripheral vessel,[42,43] retrograde approaches,[44] and use of intravascular ultrasound,[45] have been reported. After BPA of all subsegmental and segmental arteries, CT pulmonary angiogram and pulmonary perfusion scintigraphy are performed again. If mean PAP remains higher than 30 mm Hg or exercise limitation persists, those imaging modalities would help to find missed lesions and plan additional BPA. If there is no suitable lesion for BPA, uptitration of riociguat is the treatment of choice. Some other potential options, such as macitentan,[10] selexipag,[11] and subcutaneous treprostinil,[46] have been reported for CTEPH with positive results.

SUMMARY

Since the first BPA was reported in the 1980s, strategies to establish safety of BPA have been sought worldwide, which have reduced complications of reperfusion pulmonary edema and decreased BPA-related mortality to almost 0%. The long-term outcome of inoperable CTEPH has also shown dramatic improvement, with a 5-year survival rate of 90%, which is comparable to operable CTEPH. Future studies will continue to address unresolved issues, including strategies to treat refractory lesions, such as chronic total occlusions and tortuous lesions, and strategies to treat patients with chronic thromboembolic disease who remain exercise intolerant.

CLINICS CARE POINTS

- Chronic thromboembolic pulmonary hypertension occurs as a late complication in 4% of patients after acute pulmonary thromboembolism, owing to incomplete clot dissolution in the pulmonary artery.
- Five-year survival rate of chronic thromboembolic pulmonary hypertension with anticoagulation alone is less than 50% when mean pulmonary arterial pressure is above 30 mm Hg.
- Forty percent of the patients are not candidates for pulmonary endarterectomy, which is the treatment of choice, because of lesion location or age.
- Balloon pulmonary angioplasty, a catheter-based intervention, is used worldwide for the treatment of inoperable chronic thromboembolic pulmonary hypertension.
- Reperfusion pulmonary edema is a complication of balloon pulmonary angioplasty, same as pulmonary endarterectomy. However, staged balloon pulmonary angioplasty using different balloon sizes for mean baseline PAP ≥35 mm Hg and <35 mm Hg promises safe and effective treatment.
- Five-year survival rate after balloon pulmonary angioplasty for inoperable chronic thromboembolic pulmonary hypertension is 90%, comparable to that for operable chronic thromboembolic pulmonary hypertension.

DISCLOSURE

All authors declared no potential conflict of interest.

ACKNOWLEDGMENTS

This work was partly supported by JSPS KAKENHI Grant-in-Aid for Early-Career Scientists (grant number JP20K17120).

REFERENCES

1. Kim NH, Delcroix M, Jais X, et al. Chronic thromboembolic pulmonary hypertension. Eur Respir J 2019;53(1):1801915.
2. Simonneau G, Montani D, Celermajer DS, et al. Haemodynamic definitions and updated clinical classification of pulmonary hypertension. Eur Respir J 2019;53(1):1801913.

3. Delcroix M, Torbicki A, Gopalan D, et al. ERS statement on chronic thromboembolic pulmonary hypertension. Eur Respir J 2021;57(6):2002828.

4. Lewczuk J, Piszko P, Jagas J, et al. Prognostic factors in medically treated patients with chronic pulmonary embolism. Chest 2001;119(3):818–23.

5. Pepke-Zaba J, Delcroix M, Lang I, et al. Chronic thromboembolic pulmonary hypertension (CTEPH): results from an international prospective registry. Circulation 2011;124(18):1973–81.

6. Feinstein JA, Goldhaber SZ, Lock JE, et al. Balloon pulmonary angioplasty for treatment of chronic thromboembolic pulmonary hypertension. Circulation 2001;103(1):10–3.

7. Mizoguchi H, Ogawa A, Munemasa M, et al. Refined balloon pulmonary angioplasty for inoperable patients with chronic thromboembolic pulmonary hypertension. Circ Cardiovasc Interv 2012;5(6):748–55.

8. Ogawa A, Matsubara H. Balloon Pulmonary Angioplasty: A treatment option for inoperable patients with chronic thromboembolic pulmonary hypertension. Frontiers in Cardiovascular Medicine 2014;2:4.

9. Ghofrani HA, D'Armini AM, Grimminger F, et al. Riociguat for the treatment of chronic thromboembolic pulmonary hypertension. N Engl J Med 2013; 369(4):319–29.

10. Ghofrani HA, Simonneau G, D'Armini AM, et al. Macitentan for the treatment of inoperable chronic thromboembolic pulmonary hypertension (MERIT-1): results from the multicentre, phase 2, randomised, double-blind, placebo-controlled study. Lancet Respir Med 2017;5(10):785–94.

11. Ogo T, Shimokawahara H, Kinoshita H, et al. Selexipag for the treatment of chronic thromboembolic pulmonary hypertension. Eur Respir J 2022;60(1):2101694.

12. Fukuda K, Date H, Doi S, et al. Japanese Circulation Society and the Japanese Pulmonary Circulation and Pulmonary Hypertension Society Joint Working Group. Guidelines for the Treatment of Pulmonary Hypertension (JCS 2017/JPCPHS 2017). Circ J 2019;83(4):842–945.

13. Swietlik EM, Ruggiero A, Fletcher AJ, et al. Limitations of resting haemodynamics in chronic thromboembolic disease without pulmonary hypertension. Eur Respir J 2019;53(1):1801787.

14. Kikuchi H, Goda A, Takeuchi K, et al. Exercise intolerance in chronic thromboembolic pulmonary hypertension after pulmonary angioplasty. Eur Respir J 2020;56(1):1901982.

15. Inami T, Kataoka M, Kikuchi H, et al. Balloon pulmonary angioplasty for symptomatic chronic thromboembolic disease without pulmonary hypertension at rest. Int J Cardiol 2019;289:116–8.

16. Voorburg JA, Cats VM, Buis B, et al. Balloon angioplasty in the treatment of pulmonary hypertension caused by pulmonary embolism. Chest 1988;94(6): 1249–53.

17. Ogawa A, Satoh T, Fukuda T, et al. Balloon pulmonary angioplasty for chronic thromboembolic pulmonary hypertension: results of a multicenter registry. Circ Cardiovasc Qual Outcomes 2017;10(11):e004029.

18. Olsson KM, Wiedenroth CB, Kamp JC, et al. Balloon pulmonary angioplasty for inoperable patients with chronic thromboembolic pulmonary hypertension: the initial German experience. Eur Respir J 2017;49(6):1602409.

19. Brenot P, Jais X, Taniguchi Y, et al. French experience of balloon pulmonary angioplasty for chronic thromboembolic pulmonary hypertension. Eur Respir J 2019;53(5):1802095.

20. Cale R, Ferreira F, Pereira AR, et al. Safety and efficacy of balloon pulmonary angioplasty in a Portuguese pulmonary hypertension expert center. Rev Port Cardiol 2021;40(10):727–37.

21. Hoole SP, Coghlan JG, Cannon JE, et al. Balloon pulmonary angioplasty for inoperable chronic thromboembolic pulmonary hypertension: the UK experience. Open Heart 2020;7(1):e001144.

22. Inami T, Kataoka M, Shimura N, et al. Pulmonary edema predictive scoring index (PEPSI), a new index to predict risk of reperfusion pulmonary edema and improvement of hemodynamics in percutaneous transluminal pulmonary angioplasty. JACC Cardiovasc Interv 2013;6(7):725–36.

23. Inami T, Kataoka M, Shimura N, et al. Pressure-wire-guided percutaneous transluminal pulmonary angioplasty: a breakthrough in catheter-interventional therapy for chronic thromboembolic pulmonary hypertension. JACC Cardiovasc Interv 2014;7(11): 1297–306.

24. Kataoka M, Inami T, Kawakami T, et al. Balloon pulmonary angioplasty (percutaneous transluminal pulmonary angioplasty) for chronic thromboembolic pulmonary hypertension: A Japanese perspective. JACC Cardiovasc Interv 2019;12(14):1382–8.

25. Lang I, Meyer BC, Ogo T, et al. Balloon pulmonary angioplasty in chronic thromboembolic pulmonary hypertension. Eur Respir Rev 2017; 26(143):160119.

26. Cory RA, Valentine EJ. Varying patterns of the lobar branches of the pulmonary artery. A study of 524 lungs and lobes seen at operation of 426 patients. Thorax 1959;14:267–80.

27. Kandathil A, Chamarthy M. Pulmonary vascular anatomy & anatomical variants. Cardiovasc Diagn Ther 2018;8(3):201–7.

28. Nagashima T, Shimizu K, Ohtaki Y, et al. An analysis of variations in the bronchovascular pattern of the right upper lobe using three-dimensional CT angiography and bronchography. Gen Thorac Cardiovasc Surg 2015;63(6):354–60.

29. Yamashita H. Variations in the Pulmonary Segments and the Bronchovascular Trees. Roentogenologic Anatomy of the Lung 1978;70–107.

30. Gao C, Xu WZ, Li ZH, et al. Analysis of bronchial and vascular patterns in left upper lobes to explore the genesis of mediastinal lingular artery and its influence on pulmonary anatomical variation. J Cardiothorac Surg 2021;16(1):306.

31. Murota M, Yamamoto Y, Satoh K, et al. An analysis of anatomical variations of the left pulmonary artery of the interlobar portion for lung resection by three-dimensional CT pulmonary angiography and thin-section images. Jpn J Radiol 2020;38(12):1158–68.

32. Riedel M, Stanek V, Widimsky J, et al. Longterm follow-up of patients with pulmonary thromboembolism. Late prognosis and evolution of hemodynamic and respiratory data. Chest 1982;81(2):151–8.

33. Delcroix M, Lang I, Pepke-Zaba J, et al. Long-term outcome of patients with chronic thromboembolic pulmonary hypertension: results from an international prospective registry. Circulation 2016;133(9):859–71.

34. Hosokawa K, Abe K, Oi K, et al. Negative acute hemodynamic response to balloon pulmonary angioplasty does not predicate the long-term outcome in patients with chronic thromboembolic pulmonary hypertension. Int J Cardiol 2015;188:81–3.

35. Nagayoshi S, Ogawa A, Matsubara H. Spontaneous enlargement of pulmonary artery after successful balloon pulmonary angioplasty in a patient with chronic thromboembolic pulmonary hypertension. EuroIntervention 2016;12(11):e1435.

36. Kawakami T, Ogawa A, Miyaji K, et al. Novel angiographic classification of each vascular lesion in chronic thromboembolic pulmonary hypertension based on selective angiogram and results of balloon pulmonary angioplasty. Circ Cardiovasc Interv 2016;9(10):e003318.

37. D'Armini AM, Morsolini M, Mattiucci G, et al. Pulmonary endarterectomy for distal chronic thromboembolic pulmonary hypertension. J Thorac Cardiovasc Surg 2014;148(3):1005–11, 12 e1-2; discussion 11-2.

38. Cannon JE, Su L, Kiely DG, et al. Dynamic risk stratification of patient long-term outcome after pulmonary endarterectomy: results from the United Kingdom national cohort. Circulation 2016;133(18):1761–71.

39. Jais X, Brenot P, Bouvaist H, et al. BPA and Riociguat for the Management of Inoperable CTEPH: Results of the Extension Study Following the RACE Randomized Controlled Trial (RCT). Am J Respir Crit Care Med 2019;203:A1182.

40. Kawakami T, Matsubara H, Abe K, et al. Multicentre randomised controlled trial of balloon pulmonary angioplasty and riociguat in patients with chronic thromboembolic pulmonary hypertension: protocol for the MR BPA study. BMJ Open 2020;10(2):e028831.

41. Lau EM, Manes A, Celermajer DS, et al. Early detection of pulmonary vascular disease in pulmonary arterial hypertension: time to move forward. Eur Heart J 2011;32(20):2489–98.

42. Kawakami T, Kataoka M, Yamada Y, et al. Impact of CT-guided balloon pulmonary angioplasty with identification of pulmonary arterial structures distal to target lesions. EuroIntervention 2015;11(7):e1–2.

43. Hosokawa K, Abe K, Yamasaki Y, et al. A multistage strategy of perfusion SPECT and CT pulmonary angiogram in balloon pulmonary angioplasty for totally occluded lesions. EuroIntervention 2021;17(2):e167–8.

44. Kawakami T, Kataoka M, Arai T, et al. Retrograde approach in balloon pulmonary angioplasty: useful novel strategy for chronic total occlusion lesions in pulmonary arteries. JACC Cardiovasc Interv 2016;9(2):e19–20.

45. Pereira AR, Cale R, Ferreira F, et al. Balloon pulmonary angioplasty of a chronic total occlusion: procedure guided by intravascular ultrasound. JACC Cardiovasc Interv 2021;14(3):e23–5.

46.. Sadushi-Kolici R, Jansa P, Kopec G, et al. Subcutaneous treprostinil for the treatment of severe non-operable chronic thromboembolic pulmonary hypertension (CTREPH): a double-blind, phase 3, randomised controlled trial. Lancet Respir Med 2019;7(3):239–48.

The Evolution of Pulmonary Artery Denervation for Treatment of Pulmonary Arterial Hypertension

Manasi Tannu, MD, MPH, Richard A. Krasuski, MD*

KEYWORDS

- Interventional cardiology • Pulmonary arterial hypertension • Pulmonary artery denervation
- Pulmonary hypertension

KEY POINTS

- Pulmonary arterial hypertension is a progressive, life-limiting disease with few therapeutic interventions beyond triple medical therapy and lung transplantation.
- Pulmonary artery (PA) denervation is a minimally-invasive intervention that reduces pulmonary vascular resistance through ablation of sympathetic nerve fibers and baroreceptors at the main PA bifurcation.
- Preliminary animal and clinical studies have demonstrated positive effects on short-term hemodynamics. However, future studies are needed to determine the ideal timing and efficacy of intervention before integration into standard care.

INTRODUCTION

Pulmonary arterial hypertension (PAH) is a progressive, life-limiting disease that affects an estimated 10.6 per 1 million adults in the United States.[1] Despite medical therapy, PAH has a poor prognosis, with a 3-year survival rate of 68% and a 7-year survival rate of 49%.[2] Patients often present late in their disease course due to lack of access to care, suboptimal medication compliance, and delayed physician recognition.[3] For example, over 20% of patients in the modern REVEAL Registry experienced symptoms for > 2 years before PAH was recognized.[3] The consequences of severe PAH are detrimental and include right heart failure with circulatory collapse, respiratory failure, and ultimately death. In PAH patients with right heart failure, in-hospital mortality is 14% and increases dramatically to 48% once the disease has progressed to hemodynamic compromise.[4] Given the significant morbidity and mortality, many efforts have been dedicated to elucidate the underlying molecular physiology of PAH, improve therapeutic targets, and mitigate clinical progression. In this article, we aim to discuss the current management of PAH, detail the pathophysiology of autonomic dysregulation, describe minimally-invasive techniques for pulmonary artery denervation (PADN), review the current literature in animal and human trials, and explore future research directions.

Current Management of Pulmonary Arterial Hypertension

PAH is a disease of the pulmonary arterioles in which pathologic vascular remodeling leads to a progressive increase in pulmonary vascular resistance (PVR). Increased PVR results in right ventricular pressure overload. Without treatment, the right ventricle cannot overcome high pulmonary pressures, resulting in hemodynamic compromise and eventually death.

Division of Cardiology, Duke University Health System, DUMC 3012, Durham, NC 27710, USA
* Corresponding author.
E-mail address: richard.krasuski@duke.edu

Intervent Cardiol Clin 12 (2023) 381–391
https://doi.org/10.1016/j.iccl.2023.03.005
2211-7458/23/© 2023 Elsevier Inc. All rights reserved.

Abbreviations	
MPA	Main Pulmonary Artery
PA	Pulmonary Artery
PAH	Pulmonary Arterial Hypertension
PADN	Pulmonary Artery Denervation
PVR	Pulmonary Vascular Resistance
RDN	Renal Artery Denervation
RFA	Radiofrequency Ablation
6MWD	6 Minute Walk Distance
WU	Wood units
HEU	high-energy endovascular ultrasound
TIVUS	Therapeutic Intravascular Ultrasound
mPAP	mean pulmonary artery pressure
RV	right ventricular
PH	pulmonary hypertension
WHO	World Health Organization

Pathologic pulmonary vascular remodeling is caused by a combination of vasoconstriction, smooth muscle cell proliferation and thrombosis.[5] These changes are the result of an imbalance between vasodilators (prostacyclin, nitric oxide, vasoactive intestinal peptide), vasoconstrictors (thromboxane A2, endothelin, serotonin), mitogenic factors, growth factors, and thrombotic factors.[6] Genetic influences may also predispose to PAH, leading to abnormal clotting, endothelial cell production, and platelet aggregation. Pathologic genes include bone morphogenic protein receptor type 2, present in ~25% of idiopathic PAH, as well as genes coding for the serotonin transporter (linked to pulmonary artery hypertrophy) and endoglin (involved in vasculogenesis).[5,7]

Current medical therapies mostly aim to correct the imbalance of vasoconstrictors and vasodilators, while non-pharmaceutical interventions offload the right ventricle and enhance cardiac output. United States Food and Drug Administration-approved medications include modulators of vasoconstriction such as endothelial receptor antagonists (bosentan, ambrisentan, macitentan) and vasodilation such as prostanoids (epoprostenol, iloprost, tropostinil) and drugs that target the nitric oxide cascade, including phosphodiesterase-5 inhibitors (sildenafil, tadalafil) and guanylate cyclase stimulators (riociguat).[6] These drugs have demonstrated improvement in functional capacity, decreased hospitalizations, and possibly improved survival.[6,8] However, many patients have an inadequate response to treatment, fail to reach therapeutic targets, and do not maintain a sustained clinical response.[2] When medical management fails, non-pharmaceutical offloading of the right ventricle can be achieved by the creation of a pulmonary-to-systemic shunt through an atrial septostomy[9] or a Potts shunt,[10] which connects the descending aorta and left PA. Ultimately, definitive treatment of refractory disease may involve lung transplantation with possible bridging mechanical circulatory support, and palliative or hospice care.

Advanced understanding of the cellular and molecular mechanisms of PAH has led to new potential therapeutic targets. The autonomic nervous system is highly active in patients with PAH and various minimally-invasive techniques have been proposed as potential modulators, including sympathetic ganglion blockade, catheter-based renal artery denervation (RDN), and PADN.

RDN first surfaced in 2009 in a proof-of-concept publication, which showed that radiofrequency energy, delivered by a catheter in the renal artery, could lower systemic systolic blood pressure by an average of 5 mm Hg.[11] It was later proposed as a therapeutic intervention for PAH through reduction in renin-angiotensin-aldosterone system activation. However, the enthusiasm for RDN waned after the randomized controlled trial, Sympathetic Renal Denervation in Refractory Hypertertension(SYMPLICITY HTN-3),_showed no significant reduction in blood pressure after 6 months of follow-up.[12]

At the height of excitement for RDN, a few small studies assessed its effect on PAH. In a porcine model, RDN showed a significant drop in diastolic PA pressure and PVR, but subsequent pathologic investigation revealed frequent intimal vascular dissections, thrombosis, and a renal parenchymal hemorrhage.[13] Due to the potentially high risk of complications and lack of conclusive clinical benefit, the investigation into RDN for PAH has fallen out of favor. In lieu of renal denervation, the direct autonomic regulation of the pulmonary vasculature has attracted attention as a therapeutic target. This interest culminated in several animal and human trials to assess the safety and efficacy of PADN (Tables 1 and 2).

Anatomy and Autonomic Regulation of Pulmonary Vasculature

The pulmonary plexus is comprised of sympathetic, parasympathetic, and sensory nerve fibers. Sympathetic nerves that supply the pulmonary vessels arise from nerve cell bodies in the middle and inferior cervical ganglia, the first five thoracic ganglia, and the satellite ganglia.[14] At the carina, post-ganglionic fibers meet parasympathetic nerve fibers to form the anterior and posterior plexi. Nerve fibers from these plexi then enter the lungs to form a periarterial plexus, which innervates the pulmonary vascular tree, and a peribronchial plexus, which innervates the bronchial tree (Fig. 1).[14] Stimulation of these sympathetic nerves induces an increase in perfusion pressure and PVR.[14] Patients with idiopathic PAH have raised plasma levels of norepinephrine,[15,16] greater muscle sympathetic nerve activity,[17,18] and increased vessel sympathetic nerve endings,[19] suggesting an important role of the autonomic nervous system in the pathophysiology of PAH.

In addition to sympathetic nerve fibers, baroreceptors have been reported at the bifurcation of the main pulmonary artery (MPA). These pulmo-pulmonary receptors were first described by Osorio and Russek in 1962, when they noted that balloon distention of the MPA in canine models induced vasoconstriction of distal pulmonary arterioles. They hypothesized that afferent fibers of the baroreceptor lay in the adventitia of larger pulmonary vessels, while efferent fibers resided in the muscle layer; thus, PA distension induced a reflex vasoconstriction.[20] Surgical vagotomy did not alleviate the elevated PA pressure, so the afferent and efferent fibers were presumed to be independent of the vagus nerve.[20] These findings were later confirmed in

1980 by Juratsch and colleagues, who showed that distention of MPA-excited stretch-receptors near the MPA bifurcation caused acute elevation of pulmonary pressure. Investigators also successfully decreased the mean pulmonary artery pressure (mPAP) in a canine model with surgical and chemical denervation of the PA.[21] These studies formed the basis for pursuing denervation of the pulmonary autonomic system as treatment for PAH.

Pre-clinical Animal Trials of Pulmonary Artery Denervation

PADN is a catheter-based technique designed to ablate both the baroreceptors and sympathetic adrenergic fibers near the MPA. By targeted ablation, PADN modulates overactivation of the sympathetic nervous system and baroreceptor-mediated vasoconstriction, which appear universal in PAH.

The first published trial of PADN was a case series of Mongolian dogs from China in 2013. Chen and colleagues induced acute pulmonary hypertension by balloon-occlusion of the left pulmonary interlobar artery. PADN was performed at the MPA bifurcation using a radiofrequency ablation (RFA) technique with subsequent complete resolution of PH.[22] No improvement was seen when PADN was performed distal to the PA bifurcation, confirming prior findings that the afferent and efferent fibers of the baroreceptors were localized to the bifurcation.

In 2015, PADN was performed in porcine models of PH induced by thromboxane A2-mediated vasoconstriction. After PADN, there was a reduction in mPAP and PVR with a concomitant increase in cardiac output.[23] On histologic analysis, the number of radiofrequency ablation lesions correlated with hemodynamic response, suggesting a dose-dependent improvement in pulmonary hemodynamics.[23]

In 2015, a sham-controlled trial in canines showed that PADN not only improved cardiac output and mPAP, but histologic samples also demonstrated permanent sympathetic nerve injury and reduced muscularization of small PA branches, suggesting attenuation of adverse remodeling.[24] Histologic stains of rat models after PADN have also demonstrated upregulation of β-adrenoreceptors and downregulation of α-adrenoreceptors, indicating a possible long-term decrease in sympathetic nervous system overactivation.[25]

Unfortunately, these promising results have not been replicated in all animal models. Garcia-Lunar and colleagues induced chronic post-capillary pulmonary hypertension with pulmonary

Table 1
Pre-clinical animal trials of pulmonary artery denervation in pulmonary hypertension

Author	Study Type	Sample Size (PADN/Controls)	PH Type	Follow-up	Treatment	Outcomes Studied	Conclusion
Pre-Clinical Trials							
Juratsch et al,[21] 1980	Prospective case series	13/-	Canine, balloon inflation in MPA	24 h	Surgical or chemical denervation	Invasive hemodynamics	• ↓mPAP • No effect from cervical vagotomy
Chen et al,[22] 2013	Prospective case series	20/-	Canine, balloon inflation in pulmonary distal basal trunk or interlobar artery occlusion	Acute	Percutaneous PADN (7.5 F catheter with circular tip, 10 electrodes, fluoroscopy guided RFA)	Invasive hemodynamics	• ↓mPAP, ↓sPAP, ↓dPAP • No adverse outcomes • Improvements only when PADN at MPA bifurcation
Rothman et al,[23] 2015	Prospective non-randomized, sham-controlled	5/3	Porcine, TXA2 vasoconstriction	Acute	Percutaneous PADN (6 Fr spiral catheter, 1 electrode fluoroscopy guided RFA)	Invasive hemodynamics Histologic staining	• Microscopic intimal disruption, reduced medial layer thickness, altered adventitial architecture. Extent of ablation depended on wall thickness. Larger PA had minimal histologic damage
Zhou et al,[24] 2015	Prospective randomized, sham-controlled	10/10 (SN substudy 20/15)	Canine, intra-atrial N-dimethylacetamide or DHMCT	14 wk	Percutaneous PADN (7 Fr catheter, fluoroscopy guided RFA)	Hemodynamics, PA remodeling, SN injury, SN conduction velocity (SNCV)	• ↓mPAP, RAP, ↑CO, ↓RV hypertrophy • ↓ muscularization of small PAs • ↓ SNCV, axon diameter, myelin sheath thickness

Study	Design	N	Model	Time point	Intervention	Measures	Findings
Zhang et al,[25] 2018	Prospective, randomized, sham-controlled	6/7	Rat, supracoronary aortic banding (Group II PH)	4 wk, 6 mo	Surgical or chemical denervation	Hemodynamics, echocardiography, histologic staining	• Improved PA hemodynamics and RV contractile function • ↑β-adrenoreceptor, ↓α-adrenoreceptor expression
Huang et al,[41] 2019	Prospective, randomized, sham-controlled	10/10	Rat, IV monocrotaline	2 wk	Surgical PADN	Hemodynamics, histologic staining, plasma neurohormone, cytokine and receptor levels, exercise tolerance	• ↓mPAP, ↓PA and RV remodeling, ↑RV function • ↓expression of neurohormone receptor levels
Garcia-Lunar et al,[26] 2019	Prospective, randomized sham-controlled	6/6	Porcine, pulmonary vein binding (Group II PH)	3 mo	Surgical and percutaneous PADN	Hemodynamics, histologic staining, plasma neurohormone levels	• Surgical: ↔mPAP, ↔PVR, ↔RV function, ↔RV anatomy • Percutaneous: only focal damage to adventitia fibers compared with transmural PA lesion from surgical PADN

Table 2
Clinical trials of pulmonary artery denervation in patients with pulmonary hypertension

Author/Year of Publication	Study Type	Sample Sizes (PADN/control)	PH Type	Follow-up	Treatment	Outcomes Studied	Conclusion
Clinical Trials							
Chen et al,[29] 2013 (PADN-1)	Non-randomized, non-blinded, controlled phase I trial	13/8	IPAH	3 mo	Percutaneous PADN (RFA)	Hemodynamics, functional capacity, adverse events	• ↓mPAP, ↓sPAP, ↑PA compliance, ↑6MWD • No adverse events, chest pain during procedure
Chen et al,[31] 2015	Open-label phase II trial	66/-	Group I PH (PAH) Group II PH Group IV PH	1 y	Percutaneous PADN (RFA)	Hemodynamics, functional capacity, biochemical markers, echocardiography	• ↓mPAP, ↓sPAP, ↑PA compliance, ↑6MWD • Outcomes persisted at 1 y follow-up—71% chest pain during procedure • No adverse events
Zhang et al,[42] 2019 (PADN-5)	Randomize, sham-controlled trial	48/50	Group I and Group II PH	6 mo	Percutaneous PADN (RFA)	Hemodynamics, functional capacity, adverse events	• ↓mPAP, ↓sPAP, ↓dPAP, ↑6MWD • ↓clinical worsening of PH
Rothman et al,[30] 2019 (TROPHY-1)	Open-label, non-randomized, non-controlled, multi-center	23/-	Group I	1 y	Percutaneous PADN (HEU)	Procedure-related adverse events, disease progression, mortality, 6MWD, hemodynamics	• ↓PVR, ↑6MWD • No adverse events
Zhang et al,[33] 2022	Randomized, sham-controlled	63/35	Group I	6 mo	Percutaneous PADN (RFA)	6MWD, pro-BNP, hemodynamics, clinical worsening	• ↑6MWD, ↓pro-BNP, ↓mPAP, ↓PVR • No major complications

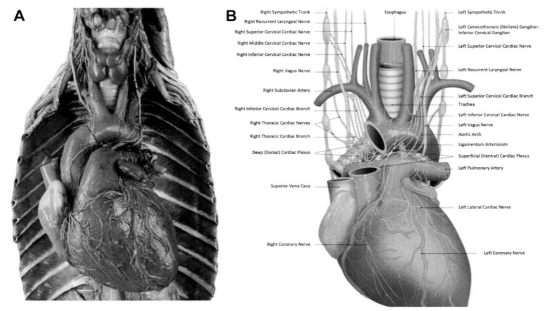

Fig. 1. (*A*) Wax mold (Courtesy of Alma Mater Studiorum University of Bologna - Sistema Museale di Ateneo| Luigi Cattaneo Anatomical wax collection. Photograph by Dr. E.A.J.F. Lakke.) demonstrating sympathetic and parasympathetic (vagal) cardiac nerves and superficial and deep cardiac plexus, (*B*) Drawing of the cardiac plexus. At the level of the heart, the sympathetic and parasympathetic nerves converge to form the superior and deep cardiac plexus. This plexus is the origin of atrial and ventricular autonomic innervation.[40] Innervation of the PA and bronchial tree.[40]

vein banding in a porcine model and then performed both percutaneous and surgical PADN. At a 3-month follow-up, surgical PADN did not show benefit in mPAP, PVR, right ventricular (RV) structure, or RV systolic function. On histologic analysis, surgical PADN created transmural lesions, while percutaneous PADN lesions showed only focal damage to adventitial fibers, suggesting percutaneous PADN to be inferior to the surgical approach.[26] It is evident from Garcia-Lunar's study of porcine models that the ideal technique for adequate denervation of sympathetic nerves depends on numerous parameters including nerve distribution, depth of sympathetic nerves, thickness of the PA wall, and the amount of energy delivered.[27]

Pulmonary Artery Denervation Techniques

PADN can be performed through a surgical approach via left lateral thoracotomy or catheter-based approaches including RFA and high-energy endovascular ultrasound (HEU).

The surgical approach was validated in porcine models using surgical bipolar radiofrequency clamps applied to the PA bifurcation and proximal left and right PA branches. Although this approach is histologically more effective at denervation, exposing PAH patients

to general anesthesia and thoracic surgery remains a risky and unattractive option.[26]

Conversely, human studies were conducted using percutaneous approaches, either with RFA or HEU. RFA is used to ablate the pulmonary baroreceptors at the level of the PA bifurcation using fluoroscopic landmarks. In the first human study of PADN by Chen and colleagues, a dedicated 7.5 F multiple-function (temperature sensing, ablation capable) catheter with a circular tip and 10 pre-mounted electrodes (separated from each other by 2 mm) were used. A baseline PA angiogram was performed to identify the PA bifurcation level and measure vessel diameter.[28] A long 8-Fr venous sheath was then delivered through the femoral vein and advanced to the main PA. The PADN catheter was advanced through the sheath, the sheath was retracted and the catheter was pushed forward to release the circular tip, which was positioned at the ostium of the left PA. The ablation parameters were programmed to a temperature >50 °C, energy of 10 W, and time of 60 seconds. Their first ablation was performed <2 mm distal to the ostium of the left PA. The catheter was then repositioned to the MPA <2 mm proximal to the bifurcation level and a second ablation was performed. Finally, the catheter was moved to <2 mm distal to the ostial right PA, and a third ablation was performed.[29]

The use of HEU for PADN was described by Rothman and colleagues using the Therapeutic Intravascular Ultrasound (TIVUS) system. The TIVUS System (SoniVie, Rosh Haayin, Israel) is a percutaneous non-contact catheter that provides a fenestrated ring of thermal effect to a depth of 10 mm, which is the expected location of the efferent and afferent autonomic nerves in the PA adventitia. The authors delivered a maximum of 18 activations to non-overlapping segments of the main, right, and left pulmonary arteries. Continuous monitoring of energy output, vessel wall distance, and temperature was used to optimize each activation.[30]

These two percutaneous techniques have shown success in phase II clinical trials with minimal procedural complications. However, the long-term efficacy and safety data remain uncertain (see Table 2).

Clinical Trials of Pulmonary Artery Denervation for Pulmonary Arterial Hypertension

Chen and colleagues published the first in-human study of PADN in idiopathic PAH (IPAH) patients in 2013 in the Pulmonary Artery Denervation-1 trial (PADN-1). PADN was performed at the level of the MPA and ostial right and left PA in 13 patients who were not responding adequately to medical therapy. The control arm comprised of eight patients who refused the procedure. At 3-month follow-up, patients with PADN experienced significant reductions in mPAP and improved 6-minute walk distance (6MWD).[22] This study was extended to an open-label phase II trial, where PADN was administered to 66 patients without a control arm. At a 1-year follow-up, there was a reduction in mPAP of 7 mm Hg and an average increase in 6MWD of 94 m. There were no serious adverse events noted, but chest pain occurred in 71% of patients during the procedure.[31]

The PADN-1 trial has been criticized for its patient population, which did not appear representative of the US PAH population. All studied patients were on long-term oxygen therapy, which is utilized by less than 35% of the current IPAH population. Furthermore, 63% of the study subjects were men, who comprise less than 30% of US PAH patients.[32] Additionally, patients were a prevalent rather than incident population (the mean interval between initial symptoms and PADN intervention was 6.8 years), which can

lead to survivor bias. Lastly, the patient population was identified as non-responders to optimal medical therapy, but their resting right atrial pressures at trial enrollment were normal, which would be considered highly unusual.[32] It is, therefore, unclear whether the study results are valid or generalizable.

More recently, an international, open-label trial at 8 PH specialty centers was conducted to assess the effect of PADN in PAH. The Treatment of Pulmonary Hypertension-1 trial (TROPHY-1) recruited patients taking dual oral or triple non-parenteral therapies who were non-responders to acute vasodilator testing.[30] The primary efficacy endpoints included change in pulmonary hemodynamics, 6MWD, and quality of life at 4 to 6 months. The authors observed a 17.8% reduction in PVR (p=0.001), as well as an increase in 6MWD and daily activity, without any significant procedural complications. The studied patients appeared to be an ideal population for a minimally-invasive, low-risk intervention, as a large percentage were already on triple therapy or had connective tissue disease-associated PAH, suggesting limited options for further therapeutic escalation or transplantation. Although these data are encouraging, the trial did not study the optimal timing or long-term impact of denervation on survival.

In 2022, a sham-controlled randomized trial of PADN for PAH was performed on 128 patients in China. Recruited patients were aged 18 to 70, had World Health Organization (WHO) Group I PAH, and were clinically stable without medical PAH therapy for at least 30 days before the trial. Per the authors, medical therapy was not withheld from patients, but rather, patients were not on therapy because it was not "clinically directed," or there were "insurance or logistical issues" that prevented them from starting therapy. Eligible patients were randomly assigned to PADN plus monotherapy with a PDE5 inhibitor or sham PADN procedure plus monotherapy with a PDE5 inhibitor. At a 6-month follow-up, PADN patients had a 33 m improvement in 6MWD, PVR reduction by 3 Woods Units (WU) (compared with 1.9 WU reduction in the sham procedure), improved RV function, and decreased N-terminal pro-brain natriuretic peptide levels.[33]

Although these short-term results are encouraging, the decision to recruit untreated PAH patients may have invited selection bias to a healthier PAH population. Despite significantly elevated pulmonary pressures (mPAP of 53.9 mm Hg and mean PVR of 10.9 WU) on baseline hemodynamic assessment, this group remained clinically stable without treatment at least 30 days before trial start date, perhaps suggesting they had a less aggressive phenotype of PAH. It is unclear how to apply these data to the general population of PAH patients. Although this study may provide valuable insight into the early application of PADN before medical therapy, it may have inadvertently studied a healthier subgroup of patients who were clinically stable despite a lack of medical therapy.

Clinical trials have also studied PADN for other etiologies of pulmonary hypertension (PH), including WHO Group II (left heart disease) and Group IV (chronic thromboembolic PH). Zhang and colleagues examined the impact of PADN on PH secondary to left heart failure. They randomized 98 patients to PADN or sham PADN and sildenafil. At 6 months, PADN was associated with a significantly lower PVR and longer 6MWD than sildenafil.[34] However, sildenafil is not considered standard therapy for Group II pulmonary hypertension and may actually worsen hemodynamics and symptoms in diastolic heart failure, calling into question the interpretation and generalizability of these findings.

PADN has also been studied in patients with residual chronic thromboembolic PH after pulmonary thromboendarterectomy.[35] The intervention arm in this study received PADN, while the control arm received a sham procedure and medical therapy with riociguat. At 12 months, decreases in PVR and 6MWD were seen with PADN compared with riociguat.[35] Although these are promising results, the study was conducted with a relatively small sample size (n = 50) and in a single-center setting. Further, riociguat was withheld from the intervention arm, which may pose an ethical challenge, as it has been independently shown to improve hemodynamics and functional capacity in a randomized, controlled study following PTE.[36] Assuming future treatment of severe pulmonary hypertension to be multimodal, an ideal study design would include riociguat in the intervention arm.[37]

Complications of Pulmonary Artery Denervation

Although PADN is considered minimally invasive, procedural complications can occur. In a sham-controlled porcine study, authors reported acute pulmonary embolism with pulmonary hemodynamic deterioration in 3 of their 16 subjects.[38] Pathomorphological examination post-PADN also revealed various micro-injuries including PA wall dissection, coagulation of media and adventitia, parietal thrombosis, and hemorrhages at the sites of RF applications.[39] In contrast, human studies have only resulted in two groin hematomas that resolved without consequence.[35] In general, the surveillance for such issues has not been well described and pathologic studies are fortunately non-existent to date.

Future Research Directions

Although preliminary data for PADN have been encouraging, the longevity of the effect remains unknown. In current human trials, the longest length of follow-up is 1 year, which may not reflect long-term consequences such as delayed re-innervation, reflex long-term vasoconstriction, or pathologic PA fibrosis. As stated above, long-term surveillance of procedural complications is also unavailable and there are no histopathologic samples from humans to identify the eventual repercussions of ablation and denervation.

More clarity is also needed on the mechanism of action of PADN, as it may have effects beyond regulating vasomotor response. Some authors have called attention to the proximity of the cardiac autonomic nerves to the pulmonary plexus. Thus, PADN may modulate both cardiac and pulmonary innervation. To this effect, negative chronotropy following the procedure has been described.[31] It is also unclear if regulation of the vasomotor response is enough to alleviate PAH. Severe, fixed, obstructive lesions have been reported commonly in the lung histology of PAH. If PADN acts solely on sympathetic-dependent vasoconstriction, it cannot alleviate these fixed-obstructive lesions, and thus, it may not have a protracted benefit on pulmonary hemodynamics.

To gain confidence with PADN as part of standard care for PAH, large-scale multi-center, randomized, sham-controlled trials with homogenous patient populations need to be conducted and replicated. To date, the study sample sizes have been small (all <130 patients), the control and interventional groups have not all been on standard medical treatment, and results have not been reproduced in multiple centers. Although PADN shows promise, carefully designed, multi-center trials are necessary to clarify the ideal timing of intervention, the true mechanism of action, and the safety and long-term efficacy in patients with PAH.

SUMMARY

PAH is a progressive, life-limiting disease with few additional therapeutic interventions beyond triple medical therapy (including intravenous prostaglandins) and lung transplantation. PADN is a minimally-invasive intervention that reduces PVR through the ablation of sympathetic nerve fibers and baroreceptors at the MPA bifurcation. Early human trials have demonstrated positive effects on short-term hemodynamics and pathologic remodeling. However, the long-term efficacy and safety of PADN remain questionable, as no studies have followed patients beyond 1 year. To gain confidence with PADN, more carefully designed, multi-center, randomized trials with reproducible outcomes need to be conducted. Future studies are needed to identify appropriate candidates, determine proper timing, and define procedural safety and long-term efficacy. Until then, PADN cannot safely be integrated into standard care for patients with PAH.

CLINICS CARE POINTS

- When treating patients with PAH, current clinical guidelines recommend referral to a Pulmonary Hypertension Center for accurate disease diagnosis, risk stratification, and optimization with one or more vasodilator therapies

- Once patients are maximized on triple medical therapy (including intravenous prostaglandins), there are few therapeutic options beyond lung transplantation or palliative care

- PA denervation may be a promising minimally-invasive treatment to improve pulmonary hemodynamics by limiting sympathetic stimulation and baroreceptor-mediated pulmonary vasoconstriction. However long-term trial data on safety and efficacy are limited

- Currently, PADN is considered an investigational treatment and not recommended for use outside of structured clinical trials

DISCLOSURE

Dr R.A. Krasuski reports serving as a consultant to Actelion/Janssen Pharmaceuticals, Bayer Pharmaceuticals, Gore Medical, and Medtronic. He receives research funding from the Adult Congenital Heart Association and Actelion and serves as an investigator for trials with Corvia, CryoLife, Edwards LifeSciences, and Medtronic. Dr M. Tannu reports no conflicts.

REFERENCES

1. Ruopp NF, Cockrill BA. Diagnosis and Treatment of Pulmonary Arterial Hypertension: A Review. JAMA 2022;327(14):1379–91.
2. Kim CW, Aronow WS, Dutta T, et al. Pulmonary Artery Denervation as an Innovative Treatment for Pulmonary Hypertension With and Without Heart Failure. Cardiol Rev 2021;29(2):89–95.
3. Brown LM, Chen H, Halpern S, et al. Delay in recognition of pulmonary arterial hypertension: factors identified from the REVEAL Registry. Chest 2011; 140(1):19–26.
4. Campo A, Mathai SC, Le Pavec J, et al. Outcomes of hospitalisation for right heart failure in pulmonary arterial hypertension. Eur Respir J 2011;38(2):359–67.
5. Humbert M, Morrell NW, Archer SL, et al. Cellular and molecular pathobiology of pulmonary arterial hypertension. J Am Coll Cardiol 2004;43(12 Suppl S):13s–24s.
6. Anderson JR, Nawarskas JJ. Pharmacotherapeutic management of pulmonary arterial hypertension. Cardiol Rev 2010 ;18(3):148–62.
7. Garcia-Rivas G, Jerjes-Sánchez C, Rodriguez D, et al. A systematic review of genetic mutations in pulmonary arterial hypertension. BMC Med Genet 2017;18(1):82.
8. Galiè N, Manes A, Negro L, et al. A meta-analysis of randomized controlled trials in pulmonary arterial hypertension. Eur Heart J 2009;30(4):394–403.
9. Law MA, Grifka RG, Mullins CE, et al. Atrial septostomy improves survival in select patients with pulmonary hypertension. Am Heart J 2007;153(5):779–84.
10. Blanc J, Vouhé P, Bonnet D. Potts shunt in patients with pulmonary hypertension. N Engl J Med 2004;350(6):623.
11. Krum H, Schlaich M, Whitbourn R, et al. Catheter-based renal sympathetic denervation for resistant hypertension: a multicentre safety and proof-of-principle cohort study. Lancet 2009;373(9671):1275–81.
12. Bhatt DL, Kandzari DE, O'Neill WW, et al. A controlled trial of renal denervation for resistant hypertension. N Engl J Med 2014;370:1393–401.
13. Vakhrushev AD, Condori Leandro HI, Goncharova NS, et al. Extended Renal Artery Denervation Is Associated with Artery Wall Lesions and Acute Systemic and Pulmonary Hemodynamic Changes: A Sham-Controlled Experimental Study. Cardiovasc Ther 2020;2020:8859663.
14. Barnes PJ, Liu SF. Regulation of pulmonary vascular tone. Pharmacol Rev 1995;47(1):87–131.
15. Nootens M, Kaufmann E, Rector T, et al. Neurohormonal activation in patients with right ventricular failure from pulmonary hypertension: relation to hemodynamic variables and endothelin levels. J Am Coll Cardiol 1995;26(7):1581–5.
16. Mak S, Witte KK, Al-Hesayen A, et al. Cardiac sympathetic activation in patients with pulmonary arterial hypertension. Am J Physiol Regul Integr Comp Physiol 2012;302(10):R1153–7.

17. Velez-Roa S, Ciarka A, Najem B, et al. Increased sympathetic nerve activity in pulmonary artery hypertension. Circulation 2004;110(10):1308–12.

18. Ciarka A, Doan V, Velez-Roa S, et al. Prognostic significance of sympathetic nervous system activation in pulmonary arterial hypertension. Am J Respir Crit Care Med 2010;181(11):1269–75.

19. Crnkovic S, Egemnazarov B, Jain P, et al. NPY/Y1 receptor-mediated vasoconstrictory and proliferative effects in pulmonary hypertension. Br J Pharmacol 2014;171(16):3895–907.

20. Osorio J, Russek M. Reflex changes on the pulmonary and systemic pressures elicited by stimulation of baroreceptors in the pulmonary artery. Circulation Research 1962;10(4):664–7.

21. Juratsch CE, Jengo JA, Castagna J, et al. Experimental pulmonary hypertension produced by surgical and chemical denervation of the pulmonary vasculature. Chest 1980;77(4):525–30.

22. Chen SL, Zhang YJ, Zhou L, et al. Percutaneous pulmonary artery denervation completely abolishes experimental pulmonary arterial hypertension in vivo. EuroIntervention 2013;9(2):269–76.

23. Rothman AM, Arnold ND, Chang W, et al. Pulmonary artery denervation reduces pulmonary artery pressure and induces histological changes in an acute porcine model of pulmonary hypertension. Circulation: Cardiovascular Interventions 2015;8(11):e002569.

24. Zhou L, Zhang J, Jiang XM, et al. Pulmonary Artery Denervation Attenuates Pulmonary Arterial Remodeling in Dogs With Pulmonary Arterial Hypertension Induced by Dehydrogenized Monocrotaline. JACC Cardiovasc Interv 2015;8(15):2013–23.

25. Zhang H, Yu W, Zhang J, et al. Pulmonary artery denervation improves hemodynamics and cardiac function in pulmonary hypertension secondary to heart failure. Pulm Circ 2019;9(2). https://doi.org/10.1177/2045894018816297. 2045894018816297.

26. Garcia-Lunar I, Pereda D, Santiago E, et al. Effect of pulmonary artery denervation in postcapillary pulmonary hypertension: results of a randomized controlled translational study. Basic Res Cardiol 2019;114(2):5.

27. Constantine A, Dimopoulos K. Pulmonary artery denervation for pulmonary arterial hypertension. Trends Cardiovasc Med 2021;31(4):252–60.

28. Chen S-L, Zhang F-F, Xu J, et al. Pulmonary Artery Denervation to Treat Pulmonary Arterial Hypertension. J Am Coll Cardiol 2013;62(12):1092–100.

29. Chen SL, Zhang FF, Xu J, et al. Pulmonary artery denervation to treat pulmonary arterial hypertension: the single-center, prospective, first-in-man PADN-1 study (first-in-man pulmonary artery denervation for treatment of pulmonary artery hypertension). J Am Coll Cardiol 2013;62(12):1092–100.

30. Rothman AMK, Vachiery J-L, Howard LS, et al. Intravascular Ultrasound Pulmonary Artery Denervation to Treat Pulmonary Arterial Hypertension (TROPHY1): Multicenter, Early Feasibility Study. JACC Cardiovasc Interv 2020;13(8):989–99.

31. Chen SL, Zhang H, Xie DJ, et al. Hemodynamic, functional, and clinical responses to pulmonary artery denervation in patients with pulmonary arterial hypertension of different causes: phase II results from the Pulmonary Artery Denervation-1 study. Circ Cardiovasc Interv 2015;8(11):e002837.

32. Galiè N, Manes A. New treatment strategies for pulmonary arterial hypertension: hopes or hypes? J Am Coll Cardiol 2013;62(12):1101–2.

33. Zhang H, Wei Y, Zhang C, et al. Pulmonary Artery Denervation for Pulmonary Arterial Hypertension: A Sham-Controlled Randomized Trial. JACC Cardiovasc Interv 2022. https://doi.org/10.1016/j.jcin.2022.09.013.

34. Zhang H, Zhang J, Chen M, et al. Pulmonary Artery Denervation Significantly Increases 6-Min Walk Distance for Patients With Combined Pre- and Post-Capillary Pulmonary Hypertension Associated With Left Heart Failure: The PADN-5 Study. JACC Cardiovasc Interv 2019;12(3):274–84.

35. Romanov A, Cherniavskiy A, Novikova N, et al. Pulmonary Artery Denervation for Patients With Residual Pulmonary Hypertension After Pulmonary Endarterectomy. J Am Coll Cardiol 2020;76(8):916–26.

36. Ghofrani HA, D'Armini AM, Grimminger F, et al. Riociguat for the treatment of chronic thromboembolic pulmonary hypertension. N Engl J Med 2013;369(4):319–29.

37. Hoeper MM. Pulmonary Artery Denervation. J Am Coll Cardiol 2020;76(8):927–9.

38. Goncharova NS, Condori Leandro HI, Vakhrushev AD, et al. Transcatheter radiofrequency pulmonary artery denervation in swine: the evaluation of lesion degree, hemodynamics and pulmonary hypertension inducibility. BMC Pulm Med 2021;21(1):418.

39. Condori Leandro HI, Koshevaya EG, Mitrofanova LB, et al. An ovine model for percutaneous pulmonary artery laser denervation: perivascular innervation and ablation lesion characteristics. Int J Mol Sci 2021;22(16):8788.

40. Zandstra T, Notenboom R, Wink J, et al. Asymmetry and Heterogeneity: Part and Parcel in Cardiac Autonomic Innervation and Function. Front Physiol 2021;12. https://doi.org/10.3389/fphys.2021.665298.

41. Huang Y, Liu YW, Pan HZ, et al. Transthoracic Pulmonary Artery Denervation for Pulmonary Arterial Hypertension. Arterioscler Thromb Vasc Biol 2019;39(4):704–18.

42. Zhang H, Zhang J, Chen M, et al. Pulmonary Artery Denervation Significantly Increases 6-Min Walk Distance for Patients With Combined Pre- and Post-Capillary Pulmonary Hypertension Associated With Left Heart Failure. JACC Cardiovasc Interv 2019;12(3):274–84.

Pulmonary Embolism Center of Excellence
Putting It All Together

Scott H. Visovatti, MA, MD

KEYWORDS

- CTEPH • Pulmonary hypertension • Pulmonary embolism • Expert center

---

KEY POINTS

- Center of excellence (COE) designations in medicine use highly variable criteria and are bestowed by a wide variety of entities.
- A well-conceived, patient-centered set of COE criteria exists and may serve as the foundation for a designation that results in an improvement in meaningful clinical outcomes.
- The highly specialized, multidisciplinary care needed to treat both acute pulmonary embolic disease as well as chronic thromboembolic pulmonary hypertension lends itself well to a center-of-excellence-based system of care delivery.
- Preexisting programs, including the Pulmonary Embolism Response Team and Pulmonary Hypertension Association Care Center accreditation program, are foundational to pulmonary embolism COE initiatives.

CENTERS OF EXCELLENCE: AN INTRODUCTION

The growing complexity of the evaluation and treatment of patients with acute and chronic pulmonary emboli requires specialized, multidisciplinary expertise based in high-volume centers. Given these needs, pulmonary embolism care seems to lend itself well to a center-of-excellence-based system of care delivery. In fact, current European Society of Cardiology/European Respiratory Society pulmonary hypertension guidelines contain specific recommendations for the treatment of acute pulmonary emboli at expert centers and the establishment of chronic thromboembolic disease (chronic thromboembolic pulmonary hypertension [CTEPH]) centers.[1,2] The purpose of this article is to review the challenges involved in defining and implementing a center of excellence (COE), the potential benefits derived from establishing a COE, current evidence-based data regarding clinical outcomes in COEs versus non-COEs in other fields of medicine, as well as the current state of pulmonary embolism COE accreditation programs.

BACKGROUND
Center of Excellence: Definition

Health-care COEs are niche programs, which assemble high concentrations of expertise and related resources aimed at providing comprehensive, multidisciplinary care in a particular area of medicine. There are no universal criteria for the establishment of, or designation as, a COE. Many COEs are defined by professional organizations, government programs, consumer advocacy groups, or even hospitals themselves.[3] Insurance companies may also establish specific criteria, as exemplified by percutaneous coronary intervention (PCI) COEs by Aetna, Cigna, and Blue Cross Blue Shield.[4] Some of the most widely known program accreditations are awarded by The Joint Commission, an independent, not-for-profit group recognized by the Centers for Medicare & Medicaid Services.

Department of Internal Medicine, Division of Cardiovascular Medicine, The Ohio State University, Davis Heart and Lung Research Institute, 473 West 12th Avenue, Columbus, OH 43210, USA
E-mail address: Scott.visovatti@osumc.edu
Twitter: @SVisovatti (S.H.V.)

Intervent Cardiol Clin 12 (2023) 393–398
https://doi.org/10.1016/j.iccl.2023.03.006

Table 1
Center of excellence distinguishing features

Feature	Description
Organization design	The manner in which work responsibilities and resources are divided and allocated to units in an institution to ensure coordination and performance, permitting mission fulfillment
Servicescape design	The collection of elements, which compose the service environment of an institution. Examples include architecture, parking, signage, equipment, technology, ergonomics, and ambiance
Personnel	Experts with a depth and breadth of qualifications are assembled via carefully planned organizational structures into collaborative, interdisciplinary teams and directed in a manner to deliver exceptional care
Medical care	Well-equipped servicescapes and expert workforces converge via effective organization designs to permit a level of medical care difficult to match outside of the COE delivery model
Marketing	Proper marketing efforts directed toward promoting the depth and breadth of services combined with excellent care delivery creates top-of-mind awareness that bolsters patient volume
Finance	Centers of excellence have the potential to improve financial performance through quality enhancements, product differentiation that increases patient volume, attainment of standards required to maximize reimbursements, and economies of scale

Adapted from Ref.[6]

Through partnerships with the Association for the Advancement of Blood and Biotherapies, the American Academy of Orthopedic Surgeons, the American College of Obstetricians and Gynecologists, the American Heart Association, the American Stroke Association, the Alzheimer's Association and the American Society for Clinical Pathology, a variety of accreditation, certification, and verification levels are offered.[5] For example, The Joint Commission/American Stroke Association offer 4 "advanced stroke certifications" for hospitals, ranging from an Acute Stroke Ready Hospital to a Comprehensive Stroke Center (CSC).

Given the variety of COE program designations, as well as the highly variable criteria used in these designations, it is helpful to identify a set of features common to COEs. One well-conceived system for designating COEs based on 6 distinguishing features is shown in Table 1. These features act as a framework for the establishment of a COE, a process that involves an initial stage of vision and plan validation, implementation of design and development stages and a final stage of completion and commercialization.[6]

Center of Excellence: Potential Benefits

There are significant potential benefits to establishing COEs. Possible clinical advantages gained by COEs include improved clinical outcomes because of a deep understanding of a specific patient population and the ability to provide individualized care using expert workforces, refined techniques, and innovative technologies.[6] COEs also benefit from being able to market their expertise, creating a "top-of-mind awareness" resulting in an increased patient volume.[6,7] Volume may also increase when large employers encourage employees to use COEs, as is the case with Walmart (which is the largest employer in the world).[3] This increased volume, combined with improved efficiency, quality enhancements resulting in the attainment of standards resulting, which maximize reimbursement, as well as the ability to lower costs by leveraging economies of scale have the potential to improve the financial performance of a COE.[6] From a personnel perspective, COEs bring together individuals with well-developed skills and expertise to form multidisciplinary, collaborative teams that provide exceptional care. Such synergistic team building pays additional dividends because it helps establish COEs as "learning organizations,"[6] a concept developed by systems scientist Peter Senge that describes institutions "where people continually expand their capacity to create the results they truly desire, where new and expansive patterns of thinking are nurtured, where collective aspiration is set free, and where people are continually learning how to learn together."[8] Given the potential benefits to be gained, it is not surprising that COE designations have proliferated throughout the health-care industry. However, significant challenges to both the definition and implementation of COEs remain, and these must be taken into account because a cohesive, outcomes-driven plan for the establishment of pulmonary embolism COE programs is developed.

Center of Excellence: Clinical Outcomes

Purported benefits to the establishment of COEs include improved clinical outcomes; however, data supporting these claims are generally lacking. For example, a study comparing 30-day risk-adjusted mortality and admission rates following PCIs in hospitals with and without COE designations for cardiac care from 1 of 3 payors (Aetna, Cigna, and Blue Cross Blue Shield) found no correlation between COE status and outcomes.[4] Another observational study comparing 3337 accredited hospitals with 1063 nonaccredited hospitals and found no difference in 30-day risk-adjusted mortality rates.[9] A comparison of centers with Primary Stroke Center certification with the more demanding CSC certification showed that these centers achieved similar care quality.[10] Findings such as these should not be taken as evidence that the COE concept is not effective at improving clinical outcomes; however, they do emphasize the importance of using clinically important criteria in the designation of COEs.

PULMONARY EMBOLISM CENTERS OF EXCELLENCE: CURRENT STATUS

The development of centers specializing in the delivery of care for pulmonary embolic disease have their foundations in preexisting initiatives including the Pulmonary Embolism Response Team (PERT) Consortium for acute pulmonary emboli and the Pulmonary Hypertension Association's Centers of Comprehensive Care accreditation for chronic disease.

Acute Pulmonary Emboli Centers of Excellence

The PERT model was developed in 2012 to improve the quality and efficiency of care for patients with intermediate-risk and high-risk acute pulmonary embolism.[11–16] A PERT is generally activated after a clinically significant pulmonary embolism (PE) is diagnosed,[17] bringing together

a diverse rapid response team that may include specialists in pulmonary/critical care medicine, emergency medicine, cardiac surgery, interventional cardiology, vascular medicine, noninterventional cardiology, interventional radiology, hematology, or noncardiac surgery.[17] In addition to providing rapid, real-time, multidisciplinary input on patient care, a PERT also facilitates internal quality assessment and improvement, multicenter research initiatives, and the generation of high-quality outcomes data aimed at addressing knowledge gaps in the field.[11] Although rapid response teams are generally thought to improve care for critically ill patients,[18,19] outcome comparisons between PERT-activated and non-PERT-activated patients have shown mixed results. For example, of 4 recent, retrospective studies that have analyzed patient-centered outcomes before and after the implementation of a PERT; 2 of these studies demonstrated a significant 30-day mortality improvement after adoption of a PERT[20,21] while 2 showed no mortality benefit[22,23] (although these relied on artificially constructed non-PERT comparator groups[21]). These findings emphasize the need for well-conceived, prospective studies that investigate the true impact of the PERT model on patient-centered outcomes.

The PERT Consortium was created to promote the adoption of the PERT model at health-care institutions across the United States, expand the body of scientific literature regarding the diagnosis and treatment of pulmonary embolism, and educate practitioners and the general public about the diagnosis and treatment of pulmonary embolism.[5] The PERT Consortium has recently announced a "PE Centers of Excellence" certification. With goals of "improving patient outcomes and safety, promoting and rapidly disseminating recent advance in technology, expanding the world's largest quality PE database, and using data-driven metrics to more quickly refine PE care,"[5] this initiative also aims to establish a "governing body for certifying competence and quality care in PE." In a recent editorial, Kobayashi and colleagues used the Elrod and Fortenberry COE criteria (see Table 1) to discuss whether the field of acute PE treatment is ready for initiatives such as the one proposed by the PERT Consortium.[24] Citing the coordinated, multidisciplinary composition of PERTs (organization design and personnel); the use of complex, cutting edge technology such as catheter-directed thrombolysis, right ventricular assist device platforms, and extracorporeal membrane oxygenation (ECMO) (medical care and servicescape

---

Box 1
European Society of Cardiology/European Respiratory Society Chronic Thromboembolic Pulmonary Hypertension Center Criteria

Prerequisite

- Fulfill criteria for a pulmonary hypertension center

Multidisciplinary Team (trained in high-volume PEA and/or BPA centers)

- PEA surgeon
- BPA interventionalist
- PH specialist
- Thoracic radiologist

Regular Multidisciplinary Meeting Topics

- Review new referrals
- Review post-treatment follow-up cases

Procedural Volumes

- >50 PEAs per year
- >30 BPA patients per year or >100 procedures per year

Medical Management

- Should manage medically treated patients

Abbreviations: BPA, balloon pulmonary angioplasty; CTEPH, chronic thromboembolic pulmonary hypertension; PEA, pulmonary endarterectomy.
Adapted from Ref.[1]

---

design); likelihood of lower length of stay due to coordinated PERT care, lower costs due to increased efficiency; and the potential for improved efficiency through clear lines of transfer to PERT centers (finance and marketing), centers with PERTs would seem to have many of the necessary COE distinguishing features identified by Elrod and Fortenberry.[6,24] The authors also suggest that acute PE COEs may benefit from integration within a "hub and spoke" model, whereby a peripheral network of hospitals transfer patients to a centralized, higher volume COE.[24] This concept is supported by a study showing a 15% reduction in 1-year mortality, a 36% reduction in 30-day readmissions, a 6% reduction in length of stay and 4% lower costs in "very high volume" PE centers (greater than 148 cases per year) compare with "low volume" centers (less than 52 cases per year).[25]

Chronic Thromboembolic Pulmonary Hypertension Centers of Excellence

As was the case with acute PE, initiatives to define and establish specialized CTEPH care

centers arose in part from a lack of adherence to expert-recommended algorithms for the management of this complex, potentially curable, disease.[26] Current guidelines recommend that all patients with suspected CTEPH be referred to an expert center for evaluation, and that these centers be based at institutions that are already designated as pulmonary hypertension centers.[2] An accreditation program for pulmonary hypertension centers was established by the Pulmonary Hypertension Association in 2011 out of concerns that expert recommended diagnostic algorithms were not being followed to completion in the vast majority of cases of suspected pulmonary arterial hypertension, as well as the observation that up to 60% of patients referred to expert pulmonary hypertension centers were already on therapy contrary to published guidelines.[5] Accredited centers aim to improve resources available to patients with pulmonary hypertension, caregivers and providers, as well as to provide practitioners with a framework for a formalized PH practice. Centers meeting rigorous criteria may be accredited as Centers of Comprehensive Care (CCC) or Regional Clinical Programs (RCP), depending on program size, ability to provide all PAH therapies and academic features of the program.[27] Since 2014, more than 80 centers have been accredited as a CCC (pediatric or adult) or RCP. Expert PH center criteria have also been established in European countries.[28]

A consensus definition for CTEPH centers is currently lacking. Early criteria (2009) were based on the capability to perform at least 20 pulmonary endarterectomies (PEAs) per year with a mortality rate of less than 10%.[29] Expert opinion now suggests that centers specializing in PEA perform at least 50 cases annually. In addition, the expansion of treatment options to include medical management and balloon pulmonary angioplasty now necessitates the adoption of an expanded criterion for CTEPH expert centers. The 2022 European Society of Cardiology/European Respiratory Society pulmonary hypertension guidelines suggest that CTEPH centers should fulfill the criteria listed in **Box 1**. These criteria have a flexibility that allows them to be implemented in systems with a single, national CTEPH center (United Kingdom and France[28]) as well as the systems with multiple centers (United States).

SUMMARY

The COE concept offers many potential benefits, including improved patient care, marketing advantages and improved financial performance. However, criteria for designating COEs are highly variable and do not always emphasize meaningful patient-centered outcomes. Thus, robust data demonstrating improved clinical outcomes at COE versus non-COE centers is often lacking. Fortunately, well-conceived criteria for the establishment of COEs are available; COE programs utilizing these criteria may be uniquely positioned to both derive the full benefits of a COE as well as gather the prospective, high-quality, patient-centered data necessary for robust outcomes assessments. The fields of acute PE and CTEPH diagnosis and treatment seem to lend themselves well to the development of a COE-based care.

CLINICS CARE POINTS

- Optimal assessment and treatment of both acute pulmonary emboli (PE) and chronic thromboembolic pulmonary hypertension (CTEPH) require a multi-disciplinary team based at high-volume centers.

- The establishment of criteria for acute PE and CTEPH centers of excellence (COE) should be based upon meaningful, evidence-based, verifiable patient-centered clinical outcomes.

- Once clear COE criteria is established and PE and CTEPH centers of excellence are established, patient outcomes should be frequently assessed to assure COE's provide improved care compared to non-COE programs.

DISCLOSURE

The author has nothing to disclose.

REFERENCES

1. Humbert M, Kovacs G, Hoeper MM, et al. 2022 ESC/ERS Guidelines for the diagnosis and treatment of pulmonary hypertension. Eur Heart J 2022;43:3618–731.
2. Konstantinides SV, Meyer G. The 2019 ESC Guidelines on the Diagnosis and Management of Acute Pulmonary Embolism. Eur Heart J 2019;40:3453–5.
3. Stefanacci MPaRG. Centers of Excellence: Criteria and Comprehensive Clinical Pathways. 2019. Available at: https://www.hmpgloballearningnetwork.com/site/jcp/article/centers-excellence-criteria-and-comprehensive-clinical-pathways. Accessed April 18, 2023.
4. Khatana SAM, Nathan AS, Dayoub EJ, et al. Centers of Excellence Designations, Clinical Outcomes, and Characteristics of Hospitals Performing Percutaneous Coronary Interventions. JAMA Intern Med 2019;179:1138–40.
5. Available at: https://www.jointcommission.org/who-we-are/who-we-work-with/our-partnerships/. Accessed April 18, 2023.
6. Elrod JK, Fortenberry JL Jr. Centers of excellence in healthcare institutions: what they are and how to assemble them. BMC Health Serv Res 2017;17:425. https://doi.org/10.1186/s12913-017-2340-y.
7. Elrod JK. Breadcrumbs to cheesecake : a struggling inner-city neighborhood sanitarium's journey to become Louisiana's largest medical center. Shreveport: R&R Publishers; 2013.
8. Senge PM. The fifth discipline : the art and practice of the learning organization. 1st edition. New York: Doubleday/Currency; 1990.
9. Lam MB, Figueroa JF, Feyman Y, et al. Association between patient outcomes and accreditation in US hospitals: observational study. BMJ 2018;363:k4011.
10. Man S, Zhao X, Uchino K, et al. Comparison of Acute Ischemic Stroke Care and Outcomes Between Comprehensive Stroke Centers and Primary Stroke Centers in the United States. Circ Cardiovasc Qual Outcomes 2018;11:e004512.
11. Giri J, Sista AK, Weinberg I, et al. Interventional Therapies for Acute Pulmonary Embolism: Current Status and Principles for the Development of Novel Evidence: A Scientific Statement From the American Heart Association. Circulation 2019;140:e774–801.
12. Kabrhel C, Jaff MR, Channick RN, et al. A multidisciplinary pulmonary embolism response team. Chest 2013;144:1738–9.
13. Provias T, Dudzinski DM, Jaff MR, et al. The Massachusetts General Hospital Pulmonary Embolism Response Team (MGH PERT): creation of a multidisciplinary program to improve care of patients with massive and submassive pulmonary embolism. Hosp Pract 2014;42:31–7.
14. Reza N, Dudzinski DM. Pulmonary embolism response teams. Curr Treat Options Cardiovasc Med 2015;17:387.
15. Kabrhel C, Rosovsky R, Channick R, et al. A Multidisciplinary Pulmonary Embolism Response Team: Initial 30-Month Experience With a Novel Approach to Delivery of Care to Patients With Submassive and Massive Pulmonary Embolism. Chest 2016;150:384–93.
16. Witkin AS, Harshbarger S, Kabrhel C. Pulmonary Embolism Response Teams. Semin Thromb Hemost 2016;42:857–64.
17. Barnes GD, Kabrhel C, Courtney DM, et al. Diversity in the Pulmonary Embolism Response Team Model: An Organizational Survey of the National

PERT Consortium Members. Chest 2016;150:1414–7.

18. Winters BD, Pham JC, Hunt EA, et al. Rapid response systems: a systematic review. Crit Care Med 2007;35:1238–43.

19. Solomon RS, Corwin GS, Barclay DC, et al. Effectiveness of rapid response teams on rates of in-hospital cardiopulmonary arrest and mortality: A systematic review and meta-analysis. J Hosp Med 2016;11:438–45.

20. Chaudhury P, Gadre SK, Schneider E, et al. Impact of Multidisciplinary Pulmonary Embolism Response Team Availability on Management and Outcomes. Am J Cardiol 2019;124:1465–9.

21. Myc LA, Solanki JN, Barros AJ, et al. Adoption of a dedicated multidisciplinary team is associated with improved survival in acute pulmonary embolism. Respir Res 2020;21:159.

22. Xenos ES, Davis GA, He Q, et al. The implementation of a pulmonary embolism response team in the management of intermediate- or high-risk pulmonary embolism. J Vasc Surg Venous Lymphat Disord 2019;7:493–500.

23. Rosovsky R, Chang Y, Rosenfield K, et al. Changes in treatment and outcomes after creation of a pulmonary embolism response team (PERT), a 10-year analysis. J Thromb Thrombolysis 2019;47:31–40. https://doi.org/10.1007/s11239-018-1737-8.

24. Kobayashi T, Young MN, Giri J. Volume, outcomes, and 'Centers of Excellence' for pulmonary embolism care. Vasc Med 2021;26:47–9.

25. Finkelstein M, Cedillo MA, Kestenbaum DC, et al. Relationship of hospital volume on outcomes in patients with acute pulmonary embolism: Analysis of a 70,000 patient database. Vasc Med 2021;26:38–46.

26. Gall H, Preston IR, Hinzmann B, et al. An international physician survey of chronic thromboembolic pulmonary hypertension management. Pulm Circ 2016;6:472–82.

27. Gray MP, Onyeador O, Wirth J. Update on the PHA Pulmonary Hypertension Care Center Network: Early Experience With the National Accreditation Program. Advances in Pulmonary Hypertension 2018;16:179–84.

28. Gibbs JS, Sitbon O. Center-based Care for Pulmonary Hypertension: A European Perspective. Advances in Pulmonary Hypertension 2018;16:170–4.

29. Galie N, Hoeper MM, Humbert M, et al. Guidelines for the diagnosis and treatment of pulmonary hypertension: the Task Force for the Diagnosis and Treatment of Pulmonary Hypertension of the European Society of Cardiology (ESC) and the European Respiratory Society (ERS), endorsed by the International Society of Heart and Lung Transplantation (ISHLT). Eur Heart J 2009;30:2493–537.

Unmet Needs and Future Direction for Pulmonary Embolism Interventions

Harshvardhan Zala, MD, MSCR[a,1], Huseyin Emre Arman, DO[b,1],
Saurav Chatterjee, MD[c,e], Ankur Kalra, MD[d,*]

KEYWORDS

• Artificial intelligence • Fibrinolysis • Pulmonary embolism • Venous thromboembolism

---

KEY POINTS

- Pulmonary embolism (PE) is the third most common cause of death after myocardial infarction and stroke.
- Because of the limitations and complications of systemic thrombolysis and surgical embolectomy in the management of intermediate-high-risk PE, interest in catheter-based therapies (CBT) has increased.
- Combined CBT approach may be an emerging option if either catheter-directed thrombolysis (CDT) or catheter-based embolectomy (CBE) regimen alone provides sub-optimal results.
- Data regarding head-to-head comparisons of various CBT options, concurrent use of other treatment modalities, and the long-term safety and efficacy of CBT devices are needed.

INTRODUCTION

Venous thromboembolism (VTE) usually develops in the deep veins of the extremities. Pulmonary embolism (PE) is a type of VTE that is most commonly (~90%) caused by a thrombus that originates from the deep veins of the lower extremities.[1] PE is the third most common cause of death after myocardial infarction and stroke.[2] It leads to significant morbidity and mortality worldwide. In 2018 alone, there were an estimated 390,000 cases of PE in the United States.[3] Furthermore, the number of hospitalizations and emergency department visits due to PE have been gradually increasing over the past decades.[4] One study reported the 30-day and 1-year case fatality rates of PE to be as high as 4% and 13%, respectively.[5] The Computerized Registry of Patients with Venous Thromboembolism registry demonstrated the 30-day mortality as 5.33% for PE.[6] With the emergence of COVID-19 disease, mortality rate from VTE had a staggering 74% overall increase.[7] In addition, patients with a history of PE continue to have a 3-fold higher mortality risk even after 30 years.[8] VTE is also known to be a recurrent disease process. Namely, in a Cochrane meta-analysis, the rate of VTE recurrence was estimated to be 13.5% with up to 24-month follow-up.[9] Patients with VTE also have long-term complications such as increased bleeding risk and chronic thromboembolic pulmonary hypertension (CTEPH). VTE has a major economic impact

---

[a] Division of Cardiovascular Medicine, Department of Medicine, Indiana University School of Medicine, Indianapolis, IN 46202-3082, USA; [b] Department of Medicine, Indiana University School of Medicine, IN 46202-3082, USA; [c] Department of Cardiology, Zucker School of Medicine at Hofstra/Northwell, Hempstead, NY 11549-1000, USA; [d] Franciscan Health, Lafayette, Lafayette, 3900 Street Francis Way, Ste 200, Lafayette, IN 47905, USA; [e] Interventional Services, New York Community Hospital, Brooklyn, NY 11229, USA
[1]These authors contributed equally to this work.
* Corresponding author. Franciscan Health, Lafayette, Lafayette, 3900 Street Francis Way, Ste 200, Lafayette, IN 47905.
E-mail address: akalra@alumni.harvard.edu

Intervent Cardiol Clin 12 (2023) 399–415
https://doi.org/10.1016/j.iccl.2023.03.007
2211-7458/23/© 2023 Elsevier Inc. All rights reserved.

Table 1
Risk stratification and treatment of pulmonary embolism

	Low Risk	Intermediate Risk (Submassive)	High Risk (Massive)
Presentation	• Normotensive • Low risk per PESI and sPESI • Normal biomarkers	• PESI class III–IV • sPESI ≥1 • Echo or CT evidence of RV strain • Positive troponin • Elevated B-type natriuretic peptide or N-terminal B-type natriuretic peptide	• Hypotension (systolic blood pressure <90 mm Hg for ≥15 min, decrease in systolic blood pressure of ≥40 mm Hg or vasopressor requirement) • Thrombus in transit • Syncope • Cardiac arrest
Treatment	• Anticoagulation: direct oral anticoagulants are preferred • Candidates for early discharge	• Anticoagulation: consider unfractionated heparin over others if any of the therapies below are possible • Systemic thrombolytic (100 mg over 2 h) • High risk of bleeding: half-dose thrombolytic (50 mg over 2 h) • Catheter-directed therapy • Surgical embolectomy • High-risk PE and cardiogenic shock: mechanical support to allow stability for thrombolysis, catheter-directed therapy, or surgical embolectomy	

in the United States annually with an estimated annual cost of $7 billion to $10 billion.[10] It has been shown that the rates of death from diagnosed PE have declined an average of 4.4% per year from 1999 to 2008. However, the mortality rate started to increase with an average of 0.6% per year since 2008.[11]

PE can be risk stratified according to determinants of presence of right heart strain on echocardiography or computed tomography (CT), hemodynamic instability, myocardial damage based on troponin elevation, and overall clot burden.[12] Risk stratification is of paramount importance, as it can guide the type of management that can be instituted (Table 1). One of the primary causes of early mortality in patients with acute PE is right ventricular (RV) failure resulting in low cardiac output and ultimately obstructive cardiogenic shock, with many deaths occurring hours to days after initial presentation.[13,14] Therefore, risk stratification guidelines focus mainly on factors that may contribute to short-term mortality such as RV dysfunction and hemodynamic instability. The American Heart Association (AHA), the European Society of Cardiology (ESC), and American College of Chest Physicians have provided guidelines for risk stratification and management of acute PE.[13,15] The categories for risk stratification provided by these guidelines are similar and include

high-risk or massive, intermediate-risk or submassive, and low-risk or stable PE.

Earlier and swift diagnosis of PE can increase patients' likelihood of survival. There have been recent advancements in the technology, specifically in artificial intelligence. Such advances can not only aid in prompt diagnosis of life-threatening PEs but also provide prognostic information, quantification of risk of PEs, and subsequent risk stratification. One example was demonstrated by Banerjee and colleagues, where a machine learning model, the Pulmonary Embolism Result Forecast Model (PERFORM), was designed to obtain patient-specific PE diagnosis risk score. PERFOM was designed to transform raw electronic medical record data into temporal feature vectors and develop a decision analytical model targeted toward adult patients referred for CT imaging for PE.[16] The main aim of this study was to arrive at a PE risk prediction that can be generalized to other populations. Their best performing model achieved an area under the receiver operating characteristic curve performance of predicting a positive PE study of as high as 0.9 (95% confidence interval, 0.87–0.91).[16] Models such as PERFORM can be used to support diagnostic decision of PEs by radiologists via CT scans. Another study by Foley and colleagues reported promising results regarding the use of automated artificial intelligence for the calculation of RV to left ventricular (LV) diameter from computed tomography pulmonary embolism (CTPE) axial images in patients with acute PE.[17] It was shown that the automated method was better at classifying patients with RV to LV ratio of greater than or equal to 1.[17] Also, it had high sensitivity in the prediction of 30-day mortality, adding important prognostic information in addition to the radiologists' report.[17] Deep learning is a subfield of artificial intelligence that is largely based on neuronal networks in which multilayer processing is used to extract progressively higher level of features from a data set. A systematic review and meta-analysis by Soffer and colleagues looked at 7 studies that reported on the accuracy of deep learning algorithm–assisted diagnosis of PE on CTPE.[18] The pooled sensitivity and specificity for PE detection by deep learning were 88% and 86%, respectively, and there was an acceptable number of false-positive cases.[18] However, included studies were retrospective in nature; therefore, future prospective studies are needed to accurately determine the true clinical impact of automated PE detection by artificial intelligence.

For many years, anticoagulation and systemic thrombolysis have been the mainstay of treatment of patients with PE. Anticoagulation alone has been an effective way of treating patients with low-risk PE. However, anticoagulation is associated with increased risk of early hemodynamic decompensation and death in intermediate- and high-risk populations.[19] Because of the increased risk of complications in such patients with anticoagulation alone, many physicians consider adjunctive therapies such as systemic thrombolysis, catheter-directed therapies, or surgical embolectomy. In patients with hemodynamic compromise, these interventions can be concomitantly used with hemodynamic support devices such as extracorporeal membrane oxygenation (ECMO).[20] Systemic thrombolysis can lower the risk of hemodynamic collapse and death in intermediate-risk patients; however, it significantly increases the risk of major bleeding.[21] Specifically, a meta-analysis involving 16 studies and a total of 2115 patients found a 9.24% incidence of major bleeding and a significant increase in risk compared with treatment with anticoagulation alone.[22] Surgical embolectomy can be considered in specific high-risk patients with cardiogenic shock, patients with massive PE who cannot receive fibrinolysis or remain unstable after its administration, or in intermediate-risk patients in whom fibrinolysis is contraindicated.[23] For patients with lower but still substantial risk of adverse events and mortality, more favorable therapies

are needed. Catheter-based therapies have gained high popularity in intermediate- and high-risk PE patients. These therapies can mitigate bleeding complications from thrombolysis. Nonetheless, catheter-based therapies in acute PE have not been studied in large well-powered randomized trials and do not have level I evidence. There are no established guidelines for such treatment modalities. **Table 2** enlists recent and ongoing prospective and retrospective studies on catheter-based management of acute PE.[24–33] PE response teams (PERT) have been established to help steer the rapidly evolving treatment paradigms. It is a multidisciplinary approach that is modeled after rapid response teams and focuses on providing patient-optimized treatment modalities, limiting costs and improving clinical outcomes.[19,34,35] Since its establishment, PERT have shown rapid success in terms of reductions in intensive care unit and hospital stays, increased utilization of advanced therapies, and lower trend of in-hospital mortality without an increase in hospital costs.[36–38] Recent guidelines from ESC and AHA have also emphasized on the incorporation of PERT into the hospital system with the need for further investigations focusing on the safety and efficacy of novel therapies and impact of PERT that will be crucial for advancement of the field.[19,39] This review focuses on currently available therapies, recent advances, and future directions in the treatment of acute PE. In this review, the authors investigate and discuss the risk stratification and definitions of the aforementioned categories of PE, and further explore the management of acute PE along with the types of catheter-based treatment options and their efficacy.

LOW-RISK PULMONARY EMBOLISM

Patients are considered to have low-risk PE when they are hemodynamically stable (systolic blood pressure > 90 mm Hg), have no evidence of RV dysfunction on imaging, and have normal cardiac biomarkers.[40] These patients are usually treated with anticoagulation and may not merit admission to hospital or can be candidates for early discharge.[41] The simplified PE severity index (sPESI) or the Hestia score can be used to aid in deciding whether such patients can be managed at home versus in the hospital setting.[13] A recent randomized clinical trial showed a low risk of adverse events among patients with no Hestia criteria or with a sPESI score of 0 who received ambulatory treatment.[42] In a randomized clinical trial by Aujesky and colleagues, patients with low-risk PE did well with outpatient anticoagulation management when

Table 2
List of prospective and retrospective studies on acute pulmonary embolism

Name of the Study	Study Type	Population	Intervention	Comparison	Outcome	Conclusion
ULTIMA 2013[24]	RCT	59 patients with intermediate-risk PE. Follow-up period was 90 d.	20 mg of tPA USAT	Unfractioned heparin	RV/LV reduced from 1.28 ± 0.19 at baseline to 0.99 ± 0.17 at 24 h (P < .001)	USAT is superior to heparin alone in patients with intermediate-risk PE in reversing RV dilation at 24 h without an increase in bleeding risk
SEATTLE II 2015[25]	Prospective case series	150 patients; 31 with intermediate-risk and 119 with high-risk PE. Follow-up period was 30 d.	24 mg of tPA USAT	No control	RV/LV reduced from 1.55 to 1.13 at 48 h (P < .0001)	USAT decreased RV dilation, reduced pulmonary HTN, decreased anatomic thrombus burden, and minimized intracranial hemorrhage in patients with intermediate- and high-risk PE
PERFECT 2018[26]	Prospective case series	101 patients; 73 intermediate-risk, 28 high-risk PE	Intermediate-risk PE treated with 28.0 ± 11 mg tPA USAT, high-risk PE treated with catheter-directed mechanical or pharmacomechanical thrombectomy	No control	89.1% (95% CI, 76.8–94.4) had decreased RV strain on echocardiogram	CDT is a safe and effective treatment of both acute massive and submassive PE.
OPTALYSE PE 2018[27]	RCT	101 patients with intermediate-risk PE	8–24 mg tPA USAT	4 different tPA protocols with different doses and durations	RV/LV reduced in all groups	Treatment with USAT using a shorter delivery duration and lower-dose tPA was associated with improved right ventricular function and reduced clot burden compared with baseline.

Study	Design	Population	Intervention	Control	Results	Conclusion
HI-PEITHO 2023 (ongoing)[28]	RCT					
FLARE 2018[29]	Prospective case series	106 patients with intermediate-risk PE. Follow-up period was 30 d	Thrombectomy with FlowTriever System	No control	RV/LV ratio decreased from 1.53 to 1.15 in 48 h ($P < .0001$)	Thrombectomy with the FlowTriever System seems safe and effective in patients with acute intermediate-risk PE, with significant improvement in RV/LV ratio and minimal major bleeding.
Wible et al,[30] 2019	Retrospective cohort	46 patients; 38 intermediate-risk and 8 high-risk PE. Follow-up period was 30 d	Thrombectomy with FlowTriever System	No control	Average MPAP reduced from 33.9 ± 8.9 mm Hg to 27.0 ± 9.0 mm Hg ($P < .001$). 71% experienced reduction in O2 requirements	Thrombectomy with the FlowTriever is safe and efficacious for the treatment of acute central, massive, and submassive pulmonary embolism.
EXTRACT PE 2021[31]	Prospective case series	119 patients with intermediate-risk PE. Follow-up period 30 d	Thrombectomy with Indigo Aspiration System	No control	Reduction in RV/LV ratio: 1.47–1.04. (27.3%). Reduction in systolic PA Pressure: 49–44.5 (9.2%)	Indigo aspiration system was associated with a significant reduction in the RV/LV ratio and a low major adverse event rate in submassive PE patients
Peliccia et al,[32] 2020	Prospective case series	33 patients with high-risk PE. Follow-up period was 1 y	Rheolytic thrombectomy with the AngioJet catheter	No control	Amelioration in functional class (from 3.3 ± 0.9–2.1 ± 0.7; $P < .001$) and an increase in oxygen saturation (from $71 \pm 15\%$ to $92 \pm 17\%$; $P < .001$).	Catheter thrombectomy with AngioJet in patients with acute massive PE and contraindications to thrombolysis is an effective therapeutic alternative that is not associated with relevant and persistent side effects

(continued on next page)

Table 2
(continued)

Name of the Study	Study Type	Population	Intervention	Comparison	Outcome	Conclusion
Toma et al,[23] 2020	Retrospective cohort	34 patients; 18 high-risk, 16 intermediate-risk	Thrombectomy with FlowTriever System	No control	CI improved from 2.0 ± 0.1 L/min/m^2 before thrombectomy to 2.4 ± 0.1 L/min/m2 after ($P = .01$). The mean pulmonary artery pressure decreased from 33.2 ± 1.6 mm Hg to 25.0 ± 1.5 mm Hg ($P = .01$).	Aspiration thrombectomy seems feasible in higher risk acute PE patients with immediate hemodynamic improvement and low in-hospital mortality.

Abbreviation: CI, confidence interval.

compared with inpatient management.[43] A recent systematic review on outpatient treatment of low-risk PE with direct oral anticoagulants reported that rates of all-cause and PE-related mortality of such patients were consistently less than 1%.[44] In addition, meta-analyses demonstrated the efficacy and tolerability of anticoagulation therapy on select low-risk PE patients.[45,46] Inferior vena cava filter can be considered in patients with low-risk PE who have contraindications to anticoagulation.

INTERMEDIATE-RISK/SUBMASSIVE PULMONARY EMBOLISM

Patients are considered to have an intermediate-risk or submassive PE if they present with clinical symptoms of PE and the sPESI score of at least 1, do not have signs of hemodynamic instability or hypotension, but cardiac imaging (echocardiography or CT) or laboratory testing for cardiac biomarkers may show RV dysfunction or RV injury, respectively. The ESC and AHA guidelines define this group of patients on similar criteria. However, AHA classifies it as submassive PE, whereas the ESC classifies it as an intermediate-risk PE.[13,15] The ESC guidelines further classify this group into intermediate-high-risk and intermediate-low-risk PE based on the presence of RV injury. RV dysfunction is identified on cardiac imaging as RV/LV ratio of more than 0.9.[47,48] RV injury is identified as pressure overload and is diagnosed with laboratory testing for cardiac-specific markers such as troponin or brain natriuretic peptide. According to ESC guidelines, a cardiac biomarker laboratory testing is done in acute intermediate-risk PE patients who have either clinical signs of PE, serious comorbidities, or positive RV dysfunction on cardiac imaging. Those with positive biomarker test are considered to have RV injury and are classified as intermediate-high-risk PE and those with a negative result are classified as intermediate-low-risk PE patients. The AHA guidelines do not have a subclassification criteria and classify any normotensive patient with either RV dysfunction or RV injury as having submassive PE. CHEST Guideline and Expert Panel Report categorizes patients in low-, intermediate-, and high-risk PE using similar criteria used by AHA.

Most of the acute intermediate-low-risk PE patients are managed as low-risk PE and treated in an outpatient setting with systemic anticoagulation.[49] However, the management of intermediate-risk PE using catheter-based therapies (CBT) has not been explored well yet because of the lack of sufficient data. With increasing requirement, various CBT devices continue to emerge and get Food and Drug Administration (FDA) approval with single-center randomized studies and large nonrandomized studies. Larger multicenter randomized controlled trials (RCTs) and meta-analyses are needed to validate the efficacy and safety of these devices.

Normotensive patients with intermediate-risk PE need to be hospitalized and those with positive troponin test should be monitored closely for hours to days due to a potential risk of hemodynamic decompensation with circulatory collapse.[49] Patients with intermediate-risk PE are initially treated with systemic anticoagulation. Rescue thrombolytic therapy is considered if the patient experiences hemodynamic instability during systemic anticoagulation.[50] However, routine use of thrombolytic therapy is not recommended in such patients, as it carries a significant risk of life-threatening bleeding, which outweighs the possible benefit from the treatment (AHA Class IIb, Level of Evidence C; ESC Class III, Level of Evidence B).[13,15] The PEITHO (Pulmonary Embolism International Thrombolysis Trial) trial enrolled 1006 patients with intermediate-high-risk PE and compared the impact of systemic thrombolysis with recombinant tissue plasminogen activator (r-tPA) tenecteplase versus systemic anticoagulation alone in terms of all-cause mortality or circulatory collapse within 7 days. They found that systemic thrombolysis significantly decreased the risk of mortality or circulatory collapse compared with systemic anticoagulation (2.6% vs 5.6%; $P = .015$), but significantly increased the incidence of life-threatening bleeding (6.3% vs 1.5%; $P < .001$).[21] The role of reduced dose thrombolysis also remains unclear with respect to both efficacy and safety. It is to be addressed in the currently ongoing phase-3 PEITHO trial (PEITHO-3), where patients with submassive PE are randomized to a reduced dose of alteplase (0.6 mg/kg to maximum of 50 mg) or placebo. This study evaluates the short-term efficacy and safety of a reduced dose of thrombolytic therapy given in addition to low-molecular-weight heparin in patients with intermediate-high-risk acute PE at 30 days, and long-term outcomes such as functional impairment, residual RVD, and CTEPH at intervals of 180 days and 2 years. Surgical embolectomy may be an alternative in select patients with intermediate-high-risk PE. However, its routine use in such patients is also not recommended.[51]

Table 3
Description of devices used for catheter-directed thrombolysis and their principals

Device Name	Image	Principal	French Size
Uni-Fuse		Standard CDT	4–5F
Crag-McNamara		Standard CDT	4–5F
EKOS		USAT (CDT)	5.4 F
FlowTriever		Manual aspiration thrombectomy (CBE)	20 F
Indigo aspiration system		Manual aspiration thrombectomy (CBE)	8 F

(continued on next page)

Table 3 (continued)			
Device Name	**Image**	**Principal**	**French Size**
AngioVac catheter	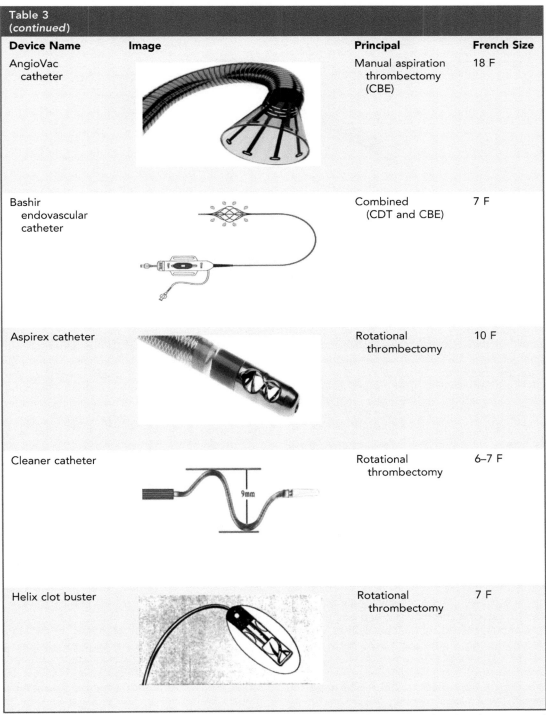	Manual aspiration thrombectomy (CBE)	18 F
Bashir endovascular catheter		Combined (CDT and CBE)	7 F
Aspirex catheter		Rotational thrombectomy	10 F
Cleaner catheter		Rotational thrombectomy	6–7 F
Helix clot buster		Rotational thrombectomy	7 F

(continued on next page)

Table 3
(continued)

Device Name	Image	Principal	French Size
AngioJet catheter	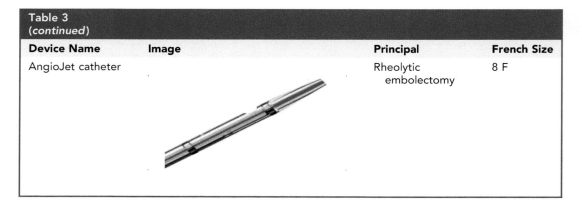	Rheolytic embolectomy	8 F

Because of the limitations of both systemic thrombolysis and surgical embolectomy in the management of patients with intermediate-high-risk PE, interest in catheter-based management has increased, with many devices emerging and getting FDA approvals with results from small single-center randomized trials.[19] Concrete results from large multicenter randomized trials to validate the efficacy and safety of these devices are still awaited. Main goal of these CBTs is to rapidly decrease the load of thrombotic obstruction in the PAs. CBTs are broadly categorized into 2 categories: catheter-directed thrombolysis (CDT) and catheter-based embolectomy (CBE).[52] These devices use various types of mechanical, pharmacologic, or combined pharmacomechanical approaches to lyse and remove thrombus from PA. Varieties of devices with their descriptions and mechanisms are shown in Table 3.

CATHETER-DIRECTED THROMBOLYSIS

CDT method uses an approach where a thrombolytic agent is administered directly into the PA via catheter. This targeted approach allows for a usage of lower dose of a thrombolytic agent to achieve similar efficacy of thrombolysis as with systemic thrombolysis and decrease the rate of major bleeding. Multiple studies have reported the use of one-fourth dose of the thrombolytic agent with CDTs compared with systemic thrombolysis.[24,25] An additional advantage of this targeted approach is that it eliminates the possibility of blood shunting toward the unobstructed artery rather than toward the artery with the obstruction, which commonly occurs with systemic thrombolysis. Uni-Fuse and Cragg-McNamara are the most commonly used CDT catheters (see Table 3).

Ultrasound-assisted thrombolysis (USAT) is another type of CDT that uses similar approach

of the administration of a thrombolytic agent directly into the PA via catheter with an additional application of local ultrasound through an additional lumen of the catheter. The addition of local application of a low-energy ultrasound facilitates the dissociation of fibrin strands to ultimately provide a more effective thrombolysis. EkoSonic Endovascular System is the only currently FDA-approved device that uses this mechanism. This type of CDT augmented with USAT is more commonly used than simple infusion catheters. Multiple trials have evaluated the efficacy and safety of the ultrasound-assisted CDTs. ULTIMA (Ultrasound Accelerated Thrombolysis of Pulmonary Embolism) was a multicenter RCT that included 59 patients of intermediate-risk PE with an RV/LV ratio of more than 1.0 on echocardiography.[24] The patients were randomized into systemic anticoagulation with either unfractionated heparin (UFH) alone or UFH and USAT. The primary outcome of the study was the difference in the RV/LV ratio from baseline to 24 hours. Safety outcomes included all-cause mortality, major bleeding, and recurrent VTE at 90 days. The investigators found that at 24 hours, USAT and UFH regimen reduced the RV/LV ratio to a greater extent than anticoagulation with UFH alone. However, there was no difference in the rate of major bleeding between the 2 regimens. In addition, none of the safety outcomes, including all-cause mortality, were significantly different at 90 days. SEATTLE II (EkoSonic Endovascular System and Activase for Treatment of Acute Pulmonary Embolism) is another single-arm, multicenter RCT that evaluated the efficacy of a USAT regimen (EkoSonic Endovascular System and r-tPA) in 119 patients with intermediate-risk PE.[25] They found that the mean RV/LV ratio decreased from 1.55 to 1.13 (mean difference, −0.42; $P < .0001$) from baseline to 48 hours after the procedure. OPTALYSE-PE (Optimum

Duration of Acoustic Pulse Thrombolysis Procedure in Acute Intermediate-Risk Pulmonary Embolism) is an RCT that evaluated 4 different regimens of doses and durations of lysis with USAT (EkoSonic Endovascular System and r-tPA) among 131 patients with intermediate-risk PE.[27] The study demonstrated a comparable reduction in the RV/LV ratio postprocedure compared with baseline. A recently concluded SUNSET sPE trial (multicenter, randomized, single-blind clinical trial comparing Standard vs Ultrasound-Assisted Thrombolysis for Submassive Pulmonary Embolism) enrolled 81 patients with acute submassive PE and compared USAT versus standard CDT (SCDT) regimens.[53] The investigators found that there was no significant difference in mean thrombus score reduction between the 2 groups (USAT group: from 31 ± 4 at baseline to 22 ± 7; SCDT group: from 33 ± 4–23 ± 7; $P = .76$). The mean reduction in RV/LV ratio from baseline to 48 hours was not significantly different between the 2 groups (USAT group: from 1.54 ± 0.30–0.37 ± 0.34; SCDT group: from 1.69 ± 0.44–0.59 ± 0.42; $P = .01$). In addition, major bleeding complications (1 stroke and 1 vaginal bleed requiring blood transfusion) occurred in 2 patients, both in the USAT group. The study concluded that the USAT for sPE may not confer additional benefits of SCDT, but larger trials using shorter lysis times (4–6 hours) may be needed.

CATHETER-BASED EMBOLECTOMY

CBE is the second broad category among CBTs and includes various types of mechanical regimens for the management of acute PE. These regimens include catheter-based thrombus maceration, rheolytic thrombectomy, and manual aspiration thrombectomy. There are different devices that use different mechanical approaches. An example of a device that uses manual aspiration thrombectomy mechanism is FlowTriever. It is a large-bore volume-controlled suction catheter, where the catheter is advanced over a guidewire and the thrombus is then manually aspirated using negative pressure.[54] This approach is effective in most of the cases. However, there is an additional functionality to the FlowTriever device. It also contains 3 self-expanding disks that fan out to entrain the thrombus and are then retracted back into the catheter. Main peripheral access for the FlowTriever device is either via femoral vein or via internal jugular vein. The blood loss during the procedure should be carefully monitored, as the aspirated blood is not recirculated back.

The FLARE study (a prospective, multicenter, single-arm RCT), which was conducted on 106 patients with intermediate-risk acute PE to evaluate the FlowTriever device, found that the RV/LV ratio was reduced by 0.39 from baseline to 48 hours postprocedure.[29] No device-related deaths were reported during the study.

Another device using the manual aspiration thrombectomy approach is the Indigo system (Indigo thrombectomy system or Indigo aspiration system). It is a smaller bore aspiration catheter, developed initially to treat embolic stroke. This device entrains thrombus and extracts it with a continuous vacuum pump. A prospective, single-arm, multicenter RCT, EXTRACT-PE (Evaluating the Safety and Efficacy of the Indigo Aspiration System in acute PE) was conducted in 119 intermediate-risk PE patients and reported that the RV/LV ratio was reduced by 0.43 from baseline to 48 hours after the start of the procedure.[31] In addition, major adverse events occurred in only 2 patients (1.7%), and 3 patients died within 30 days of intervention. Most of the patients (98.3%) did not require adjunctive fibrinolytic therapy.

AngioVac is another device that works on manual aspiration thrombectomy mechanism.[54] Multiple studies have been conducted to evaluate the safety and efficacy of the AngioVac device.[55–58] This device functions as an extracorporeal bypass circuit. It has a centrifugal pump, where blood is removed via suction cannula, filtered in the device for the removal of thrombus, and then reinfused back. Main advantages of this device include removal of a variety of intravascular obstructions, including tumor emboli, fibrin sheaths formed due to pacemaker leads, and inferior vena cava filter-associated embolism. The disadvantages include requirement for general anesthesia, large cannulas, and the technical difficulty of positioning the cannulas within the pulmonary tree. However, most of the studies that evaluated this device were single-center, small case series. A technique of manual thrombus maceration/fragmentation has been reported by Schmitz-Rode and colleagues, where a coaxial sheath and a pigtail catheter are advanced to the distal end of the thrombus and then the pigtail catheter is threaded through a side port of the sheath and rotated to fragment the clot.[59,60] There are second- and third-generation AngioVac devices with an addition of radiopaque markers, improved over-the-wire capabilities, and improved navigation with 20-degree and 180-degree angled tips. Concerns for maneuverability and right heart injury have limited the second-generation AngioVac device use in the pulmonary vasculature.[54] There are no data available yet for the use of third-generation AngioVac device in the pulmonary tree.

Rotational thrombectomy is a type of CBT that uses multiple mechanisms of CBE. It works on a principle that the catheter with an internal rotating head is inserted into the obstructed pulmonary artery segment. It creates a low-pressure zone that entraps the clot, which is then fragmented by the action of the catheter tip and aspirated into a reservoir.[54] It limits the distal embolization of the thrombus. However, the blood loss should be closely monitored, as aspirated blood is not recirculated. The devices that use the rotational thrombectomy mechanism include Aspirex mechanical thrombectomy device, CLEANER rotational thrombectomy system, and Helix clot buster. The evidence for efficacy and safety of these devices is limited to mostly case reports and case series, and none of these devices are FDA approved for use in the pulmonary vasculature.[61–64]

Rheolytic embolectomy is another broad category of CBT, which uses the Bernoulli effect to lyse the thrombus.[52,54] A high-velocity saline jet is blown through the catheter that is used to create a low-pressure zone that lyses the clots as they are entrained with fragments and aspirated to prevent distal embolization. One of the devices that uses this mechanism is AngioJet Rheolytic Thrombectomy System. The device has shown high rates of success in smaller studies but with significant complications, including death, major bleeding, bradyarrhythmias, and hemodynamic instability. The high rates of complications associated with this device may be due to release of vasoactive substances from platelets and cell lysis.[65] Based on this, the FDA has released a black box warning for the intrapulmonary use of the AngioJet device.

CDT may be used in conjunction with CBE in select cases. The use of combined CBT strategies has been limited due to lack of enough evidence, different procedure times and device costs. However, combined CBT approach may be an emerging option if either CDT or CBE regimen alone provide suboptimal results. The Bashir Endovascular Catheter system is an example of the device that uses this combined approach.[54] In this system, the catheter is threaded through thrombus, which allows for localized infusion of thrombolytic medications. The distal segment of the catheter contains an expandable basket with multiple infusion ports through which the medications are infused, and the clot is entrapped. Low-dose tPA infusion via Bashir Endovascular Catheter has been investigated in the RESCUE trial.[66] It has been shown to significantly decrease the RV/LV diameter ratio and the rate of adverse events or major bleeding when used in patients with intermediate-risk PE.[66]

The data for CBE and CDT in patients with intermediate-risk PE are encouraging. However, most of the available data are based on small, single-arm studies, which may not focus on long-term cardiopulmonary health after PE. Currently, the FLASH study, a continuation of the FLARE study with intended 500 patients and 6 months of follow-up, is underway. The study is estimated to be completed in year 2023, and the results of this study are awaited, which may shed some light on these unanswered questions.[67]

HIGH-RISK PULMONARY EMBOLISM

Patients with high-risk PE present with syncope, systemic arterial hypotension, cardiogenic shock, or cardiac arrest. The ESC defines hemodynamic instability in high-risk PE patients as systolic hypotension less than 90 mm Hg, a decrease of more than 40 mm Hg for at least 15 minutes or need for vasopressor support.[13] These patients constitute ~5% of cases but have a staggering 30-day mortality rate exceeding 50%.[68,69] Therefore, patients with high-risk PE are usually treated at critical care settings. These patients often require systemic thrombolysis, surgical thrombectomy, endovascular catheter–based treatments, and/or mechanical circulatory support. Systemic thrombolysis is the most well-studied of these treatment options and is the cornerstone therapy if bleeding risk is acceptable.[15] In high-risk PE, systemic thrombolysis is well-tolerated; in fact, it is associated with decreased risk of mortality, lower subsequent risk of developing CTEPH, and improved quality of life.[22,70] However, systemic thrombolysis, as expected, is associated with increased risk of bleeding. ESC classifies thrombolytic administration in patients with acute high-risk PE as a grade 1B recommendation, and the 2016 CHEST guidelines list it as a grade 2B recommendation.[13,71] Despite these facts, recent studies demonstrated a 22.5% in-hospital mortality associated with systemic anticoagulation and thrombolysis.[72,73] Also, systemic thrombolytic therapy is associated with significant bleeding, including a 6% risk of major bleeding and up to 3% risk of intracranial hemorrhage.[21] Therefore, there has been an emerging interest in catheter-based treatment modalities. In addition, surgical embolectomy can be preferred in patients with high-risk PE who have absolute contraindication to thrombolytic therapy, failed thrombolytic therapy, or are in cardiogenic shock that may cause death before thrombolytic therapy.[74] Of note, surgical embolectomy is considered as first-line therapy for patients with thrombus in the right heart or across patent foramen ovale (clot in transit). Recent studies have shown favorable outcomes with surgical embolectomy on select high-risk PE patients.[51,75]

There are only few studies that investigated the efficacy and safety of catheter-based management of PE in high-risk populations. Among these, SEATTLE II, a prospective case series, is the largest study that included 31 high-risk patients along with 119 intermediate-risk patients. SEATTLE II study concluded that USAT decreased RV dilation, reduced pulmonary hypertension, decreased anatomic thrombus burden, and minimized intracranial hemorrhage in patients with intermediate- and high-risk PE.[25] In addition, PERFECT 2018 was also a prospective case series that included 73 intermediate- and 28 high-risk PE patients that concluded that catheter-directed therapy is a safe and effective treatment of both intermediate- and high-risk PE patients.[26] There are a few other smaller studies that included high-risk PE patients who were treated with catheter-directed therapies, and all confirmed the safety and efficacy of this treatment modality.[30,32,33] The FLAME study (NCT04795167) is a highly anticipated large prospective cohort study that aims to evaluate treatment outcomes of patients diagnosed with high-risk PE.[76] Unfortunately, there are no completed randomized clinical trials on this topic yet.

Primary cause of death in acute high-risk PE patients is RV dysfunction. Therefore, mechanical support devices including VA-ECMO, Impella RP (Abiomed Inc, Danvers, MA, USA), the TandemHeart right ventricular assist device (TandemLife, Pittsburg, PA, USA), and Protek-Duo (LivaNova PLC, London, England) may be used to augment cardiac output, which would ultimately improve systemic circulation and oxygenation. Most of the time, these RV support devices and ECMO are inserted percutaneously, although vascular cut-down approaches may be required for select patients. Mechanical circulatory support devices should always be considered as an option for patients who have high-risk PE and present with circulatory collapse or cardiac arrest. A single-center retrospective study that compared outcomes of 60 high-risk PE patients with shock or postcardiac arrest pre-ECMO and post-ECMO demonstrated significantly increased 30-day survival after increased ECMO utilization.[77] ECMO can also be used to transition high-risk PE patients to intervention; this has multiple advantages including additional time to prepare the operating staff and room, better planning of the intervention, and reduction of hypoxia-induced neurogenic damage. A retrospective cohort study involving 56 high-risk PE patients (27 undergoing surgical embolectomy and 29 undergoing protocolized approach of triage and optimization using VA-ECMO) demonstrated that institution of VA-ECMO is an effective method to triage and optimize patients with high-risk PE to recovery or intervention.[78] Namely, more patients in the protocolized group survived to 1 year and, despite planned surgical embolectomy, many protocolized patients stabilized with anticoagulation alone. Treatment with VA-ECMO and systemic anticoagulation as a bridge to embolectomy may be an effective treatment modality.[77] However, prospective trials will be needed to further investigate this topic. In addition, in centers with no availability of ECMO, percutaneous RV assist devices can be used as a bridge to definitive therapy, such as surgical or catheter-based embolectomy.[79,80]

CONCLUSION AND FUTURE DIRECTIONS

CBT have been emerging as revolutionary modalities for the treatment of PE and CTEPH. However, the validity of the results of efficacy and safety of these therapies in intermediate- and high-risk PE and CTEPH have not yet been proven. The current evidence in the support of these devices comes mainly from single-arm studies and case series. More concrete evidence from randomized multicenter studies is required to validate the true benefits of these devices. The subdivision of intermediate-risk PE into intermediate-high and intermediate-low-risk categories and available treatment options show the importance of the ongoing need for continued research to determine optimal treatment strategies in intermediate-risk PE. In addition, data regarding head-to-head comparisons of various CBT options, concurrent use of other treatment modalities, and the long-term safety and efficacy of CBT devices are needed. Continued research in these areas will optimistically lead to improved outcomes and prognosis among patients with acute PE.

CLINICS CARE POINTS

- Patients with low-risk PE and hemodynamically stable patients with intermediate-risk PE are usually treated with anticoagulation and may not merit admission to the hospital or can be candidates for early discharge.

- Rescue thrombolytic therapy or surgical embolectomy can be considered in patients with intermediate-risk PE experiencing hemodynamic instability. However, because of the limitations of these approaches, their routine use is not recommended in such patients.

- Catheter-based therapies have recently been increasingly approved by FDA and used in patients with intermediate-risk PE.

- Catheter-directed thrombolysis (CDT) uses a targeted approach to pulmonary artery via catheter that allows for usage of lower dose of a thrombolytic agent to achieve similar efficacy of thrombolysis as with systemic thrombolysis and decrease the rate of major bleeding.

- Catheter-based embolectomy (CBE) uses an approach that causes mechanical or ultrasound-guided lysis and aspiration of a pulmonary embolus.

- Most of the data on uses of CDT and CBE are from single-arm studies and case series. Data regarding head-to-head comparisons, concurrent use of other treatment modalities, and long-term safety and efficacy of CBT devices with concrete evidence from multiple randomized controlled trials are needed.

- Patients with high-risk PE often require systemic thrombolysis, surgical thrombectomy, endovascular catheter–based treatments, and/or mechanical circulatory support.

DISCLOSURE

The authors have nothing to disclose.

REFERENCES

1. Raskob GE, Silverstein R, Bratzler DW, et al. Surveillance for deep vein thrombosis and pulmonary embolism: recommendations from a national workshop. Am J Prev Med 2010;38(4 Suppl):S502–9.
2. Horlander KT, Mannino DM, Leeper KV. Pulmonary embolism mortality in the United States, 1979-1998: an analysis using multiple-cause mortality data. Arch Intern Med 2003;163(14):1711–7.
3. Tsao CW, Aday AW, Almarzooq ZI, et al. Heart Disease and Stroke Statistics-2022 Update: A Report From the American Heart Association. Circulation 2022;145(8):e153–639.
4. Minges KE, Bikdeli B, Wang Y, et al. National Trends in Pulmonary Embolism Hospitalization Rates and Outcomes for Adults Aged ≥65 Years in the United States (1999 to 2010). Am J Cardiol 2015;116(9):1436–42.
5. Alotaibi GS, Wu C, Senthilselvan A, et al. Secular Trends in Incidence and Mortality of Acute Venous Thromboembolism: The AB-VTE Population-Based Study. Am J Med 2016;129(8):879.e19–25.
6. Bikdeli B, Jimenez D, Hawkins M, et al. Rationale, Design and Methodology of the Computerized Registry of Patients with Venous Thromboembolism (RIETE). Thromb Haemost 2018;118(1):214–24.
7. Malas MB, Naazie IN, Elsayed N, et al. Thromboembolism risk of COVID-19 is high and associated with a higher risk of mortality: A systematic review and meta-analysis. EClinicalMedicine 2020;29:100639.
8. Søgaard KK, Schmidt M, Pedersen L, et al. 30-year mortality after venous thromboembolism: a population-based cohort study. Circulation 2014;130(10):829–36.
9. Kirkilesis G, Kakkos SK, Bicknell C, et al. Treatment of distal deep vein thrombosis. Cochrane Database Syst Rev 2020;4(4):CD013422.
10. Grosse SD, Nelson RE, Nyarko KA, et al. The economic burden of incident venous thromboembolism in the United States: A review of estimated attributable healthcare costs. Thromb Res 2016;137:3–10.
11. Martin KA, Molsberry R, Cuttica MJ, et al. Time Trends in Pulmonary Embolism Mortality Rates in the United States, 1999 to 2018. J Am Heart Assoc 2020;9(17):e016784.
12. Corrigan D, Prucnal C, Kabrhel C. Pulmonary embolism: the diagnosis, risk-stratification, treatment and disposition of emergency department patients. Clin Exp Emerg Med 2016;3(3):117–25.
13. Konstantinides SV, Meyer G, Becattini C, et al. ESC Guidelines for the diagnosis and management of acute pulmonary embolism developed in collaboration with the European Respiratory Society (ERS): The Task Force for the diagnosis and management of acute pulmonary embolism of the European Society. Eur Respir J 2019;54(3). https://doi.org/10.1183/13993003.01647-2019.
14. Pengo V, Lensing AWA, Prins MH, et al. Incidence of chronic thromboembolic pulmonary hypertension after pulmonary embolism. N Engl J Med 2004;350(22):2257–64.

15. Jaff MR, McMurtry MS, Archer SL, et al. Management of massive and submassive pulmonary embolism, iliofemoral deep vein thrombosis, and chronic thromboembolic pulmonary hypertension: a scientific statement from the American Heart Association. Circulation 2011;123(16):1788–830.

16. Banerjee I, Sofela M, Yang J, et al. Development and Performance of the Pulmonary Embolism Result Forecast Model (PERFORM) for Computed Tomography Clinical Decision Support. JAMA Netw Open 2019;2(8):e198719.

17. Foley RW, Glenn-Cox S, Rossdale J, et al. Automated calculation of the right ventricle to left ventricle ratio on CT for the risk stratification of patients with acute pulmonary embolism. Eur Radiol 2021;31(8):6013–20.

18. Soffer S, Klang E, Shimon O, et al. Deep learning for pulmonary embolism detection on computed tomography pulmonary angiogram: a systematic review and meta-analysis. Sci Rep 2021;11(1):15814.

19. Giri J, Sista AK, Weinberg I, et al. Interventional Therapies for Acute Pulmonary Embolism: Current Status and Principles for the Development of Novel Evidence: A Scientific Statement From the American Heart Association. Circulation 2019;140(20):e774–801.

20. Elder M, Blank N, Shemesh A, et al. Mechanical Circulatory Support for High-Risk Pulmonary Embolism. Interv Cardiol Clin 2018;7(1):119–28.

21. Meyer G, Vicaut E, Danays T, et al. Fibrinolysis for patients with intermediate-risk pulmonary embolism. N Engl J Med 2014;370(15):1402–11.

22. Chatterjee S, Chakraborty A, Weinberg I, et al. Thrombolysis for pulmonary embolism and risk of all-cause mortality, major bleeding, and intracranial hemorrhage: a meta-analysis. JAMA 2014;311(23):2414–21.

23. Yavuz S, Toktas F, Goncu T, et al. Surgical embolectomy for acute massive pulmonary embolism. Int J Clin Exp Med 2014;7(12):5362–75.

24. Kucher N, Boekstegers P, Müller OJ, et al. Randomized, controlled trial of ultrasound-assisted catheter-directed thrombolysis for acute intermediate-risk pulmonary embolism. Circulation 2014;129(4):479–86.

25. Piazza G, Hohlfelder B, Jaff MR, et al. A Prospective, Single-Arm, Multicenter Trial of Ultrasound-Facilitated, Catheter-Directed, Low-Dose Fibrinolysis for Acute Massive and Submassive Pulmonary Embolism: The SEATTLE II Study. JACC Cardiovasc Interv 2015;8(10):1382–92.

26. Kuo WT, Banerjee A, Kim PS, et al. Pulmonary Embolism Response to Fragmentation, Embolectomy, and Catheter Thrombolysis (PERFECT): Initial Results From a Prospective Multicenter Registry. Chest 2015;148(3):667–73.

27. Tapson VF, Sterling K, Jones N, et al. A Randomized Trial of the Optimum Duration of Acoustic Pulse Thrombolysis Procedure in Acute Intermediate-Risk Pulmonary Embolism: The OPTALYSE PE Trial. JACC Cardiovasc Interv 2018;11(14):1401–10.

28. Klok FA, Piazza G, Sharp ASP, et al. Ultrasound-facilitated, catheter-directed thrombolysis vs anticoagulation alone for acute intermediate-high-risk pulmonary embolism: Rationale and design of the HI-PEITHO study. Am Heart J 2022;251:43–53.

29. Tu T, Toma C, Tapson VF, et al. A Prospective, Single-Arm, Multicenter Trial of Catheter-Directed Mechanical Thrombectomy for Intermediate-Risk Acute Pulmonary Embolism: The FLARE Study. JACC Cardiovasc Interv 2019;12(9):859–69.

30. Wible BC, Buckley JR, Cho KH, et al. Safety and Efficacy of Acute Pulmonary Embolism Treated via Large-Bore Aspiration Mechanical Thrombectomy Using the Inari FlowTriever Device. J Vasc Interv Radiol 2019;30(9):1370–5.

31. Sista AK, Horowitz JM, Tapson VF, et al. Indigo Aspiration System for Treatment of Pulmonary Embolism: Results of the EXTRACT-PE Trial. JACC Cardiovasc Interv 2021;14(3):319–29.

32. Pelliccia F, De Luca A, Pasceri V, et al. Safety and Outcome of Rheolytic Thrombectomy for the Treatment of Acute Massive Pulmonary Embolism. J Invasive Cardiol 2020;32(11):412–6.

33. Toma C, Khandhar S, Zalewski AM, et al. Percutaneous thrombectomy in patients with massive and very high-risk submassive acute pulmonary embolism. Catheter Cardiovasc Interv Off J Soc Card Angiogr Interv 2020;96(7):1465–70.

34. Reza N, Dudzinski DM. Pulmonary embolism response teams. Curr Treat Options Cardiovasc Med 2015;17(6):387.

35. Kabrhel C, Jaff MR, Channick RN, et al. A multidisciplinary pulmonary embolism response team. Chest 2013;144(5):1738–9.

36. Jen WY, Kristanto W, Teo L, et al. Assessing the Impact of a Pulmonary Embolism Response Team and Treatment Protocol on Patients Presenting With Acute Pulmonary Embolism. Heart Lung Circ 2020;29(3):345–53.

37. Rosovsky R, Chang Y, Rosenfield K, et al. Changes in treatment and outcomes after creation of a pulmonary embolism response team (PERT), a 10-year analysis. J Thromb Thrombolysis 2019;47(1):31–40.

38. Wright C, Elbadawi A, Chen YL, et al. The impact of a pulmonary embolism response team on the efficiency of patient care in the emergency department. J Thromb Thrombolysis 2019;48(2):331–5.

39. Rivera-Lebron B, McDaniel M, Ahrar K, et al. Diagnosis, Treatment and Follow Up of Acute Pulmonary Embolism: Consensus Practice from the PERT Consortium. Clin Appl Thromb Off J Int

Acad Clin Appl Thromb 2019;25. 1076029619853037.

40. Kahn SR, de Wit K. Pulmonary Embolism. N Engl J Med 2022;387(1):45–57.

41. van Es N, Coppens M, Schulman S, et al. Direct oral anticoagulants compared with vitamin K antagonists for acute venous thromboembolism: evidence from phase 3 trials. Blood 2014;124(12): 1968–75.

42. Roy PM, Penaloza A, Hugli O, et al. Triaging acute pulmonary embolism for home treatment by Hestia or simplified PESI criteria: the HOME-PE randomized trial. Eur Heart J 2021;42(33):3146–57.

43. Aujesky D, Roy PM, Verschuren F, et al. Outpatient versus inpatient treatment for patients with acute pulmonary embolism: an international, open-label, randomised, non-inferiority trial. Lancet (London, England) 2011;378(9785):41–8.

44. Maughan BC, Frueh L, McDonagh MS, et al. Outpatient Treatment of Low-risk Pulmonary Embolism in the Era of Direct Oral Anticoagulants: A Systematic Review. Acad Emerg Med Off J Soc Acad Emerg Med 2021;28(2):226–39.

45. Piran S, Le Gal G, Wells PS, et al. Outpatient treatment of symptomatic pulmonary embolism: a systematic review and meta-analysis. Thromb Res 2013;132(5):515–9.

46. Zondag W, Kooiman J, Klok FA, et al. Outpatient versus inpatient treatment in patients with pulmonary embolism: a meta-analysis. Eur Respir J 2013; 42(1):134–44.

47. Frémont B, Pacouret G, Jacobi D, et al. Prognostic value of echocardiographic right/left ventricular end-diastolic diameter ratio in patients with acute pulmonary embolism: results from a monocenter registry of 1,416 patients. Chest 2008;133(2): 358–62.

48. Meinel FG, Nance JWJ, Schoepf UJ, et al. Predictive Value of Computed Tomography in Acute Pulmonary Embolism: Systematic Review and Meta-analysis. Am J Med 2015;128(7):747–59.e2.

49. Michaud E, Pan M, Aggarwal V. Catheter-based therapies in acute and chronic pulmonary embolism. Curr Opin Cardiol 2021;36(6):704–10.

50. Marti C, John G, Konstantinides S, et al. Systemic thrombolytic therapy for acute pulmonary embolism: a systematic review and meta-analysis. Eur Heart J 2015;36(10):605–14.

51. Keeling WB, Sundt T, Leacche M, et al. Outcomes After Surgical Pulmonary Embolectomy for Acute Pulmonary Embolus: A Multi-Institutional Study. Ann Thorac Surg 2016;102(5):1498–502.

52. Meneveau N. Therapy for acute high-risk pulmonary embolism: thrombolytic therapy and embolectomy. Curr Opin Cardiol 2010;25(6):560–7.

53. Avgerinos ED, Mohapatra A, Rivera-Lebron B, et al. Design and rationale of a randomized trial comparing standard versus ultrasound-assisted thrombolysis for submassive pulmonary embolism. J Vasc surgery Venous Lymphat Disord 2018;6(1): 126–32.

54. Burton JR, Madhavan MV, Finn M, et al. Advanced Therapies for Acute Pulmonary Embolism: A Focus on Catheter-Based Therapies and Future Directions. Struct Hear 2021;5(2):103–19.

55. Donaldson CW, Baker JN, Narayan RL, et al. Thrombectomy using suction filtration and veno-venous bypass: single center experience with a novel device. Catheter Cardiovasc Interv Off J Soc Card Angiogr Interv 2015;86(2):E81–7.

56. Al-Hakim R, Park J, Bansal A, et al. Early Experience with AngioVac Aspiration in the Pulmonary Arteries. J Vasc Interv Radiol 2016;27(5):730–4.

57. Resnick SA, O'Brien D, Strain D, et al. Single-Center Experience Using AngioVac with Extracorporeal Bypass for Mechanical Thrombectomy of Atrial and Central Vein Thrombi. J Vasc Interv Radiol 2016;27(5):723–9.e1.

58. Hameed I, Lau C, Khan FM, et al. AngioVac for extraction of venous thromboses and endocardial vegetations: A meta-analysis. J Card Surg 2019; 34(4):170–80.

59. Schmitz-Rode T, Janssens U, Schild HH, et al. Fragmentation of massive pulmonary embolism using a pigtail rotation catheter. Chest 1998;114(5):1427–36.

60. Schmitz-Rode T, Günther RW, Pfeffer JG, et al. Acute massive pulmonary embolism: use of a rotatable pigtail catheter for diagnosis and fragmentation therapy. Radiology 1995;197(1):157–62.

61. Eid-Lidt G, Gaspar J, Sandoval J, et al. Combined clot fragmentation and aspiration in patients with acute pulmonary embolism. Chest 2008;134(1): 54–60.

62. Dumantepe M, Teymen B, Akturk U, et al. Efficacy of rotational thrombectomy on the mortality of patients with massive and submassive pulmonary embolism. J Card Surg 2015;30(4):324–32.

63. Barjaktarevic I, Friedman O, Ishak C, et al. Catheter-directed clot fragmentation using the Cleaner™ device in a patient presenting with massive pulmonary embolism. J Radiol Case Rep 2014; 8(2):30–6.

64. Uflacker R, Strange C, Vujic I. Massive pulmonary embolism: preliminary results of treatment with the Amplatz thrombectomy device. J Vasc Interv Radiol 1996;7(4):519–28.

65. Chechi T, Vecchio S, Spaziani G, et al. Rheolytic thrombectomy in patients with massive and submassive acute pulmonary embolism. Catheter Cardiovasc Interv Off J Soc Card Angiogr Interv 2009; 73(4):506–13.

66. Bashir R, Foster M, Iskander A, et al. Pharmacomechanical Catheter-Directed Thrombolysis With the

Bashir Endovascular Catheter for Acute Pulmonary Embolism: The RESCUE Study. JACC Cardiovasc Interv 2022;15(23):2427–36. https://doi.org/10.1016/j.jcin.2022.09.011.

67. Toma C, Bunte MC, Cho KH, et al. Percutaneous mechanical thrombectomy in a real-world pulmonary embolism population: Interim results of the FLASH registry. Catheter Cardiovasc Interv Off J Soc Card Angiogr Interv 2022;99(4):1345–55.

68. Teleb M, Porres-Aguilar M, Rivera-Lebron B, et al. Ultrasound-Assisted Catheter-Directed Thrombolysis: A Novel and Promising Endovascular Therapeutic Modality for Intermediate-Risk Pulmonary Embolism. Angiology 2017;68(6):494–501.

69. Becattini C, Agnelli G, Lankeit M, et al. Acute pulmonary embolism: mortality prediction by the 2014 European Society of Cardiology risk stratification model. Eur Respir J 2016;48(3):780–6.

70. Wan S, Quinlan DJ, Agnelli G, et al. Thrombolysis compared with heparin for the initial treatment of pulmonary embolism: a meta-analysis of the randomized controlled trials. Circulation 2004;110(6):744–9.

71. Kearon C, Akl EA, Ornelas J, et al. Antithrombotic Therapy for VTE Disease: CHEST Guideline and Expert Panel Report. Chest 2016;149(2):315–52.

72. Paranjpe I, Fuster V, Lala A, et al. Association of Treatment Dose Anticoagulation With In-Hospital Survival Among Hospitalized Patients With COVID-19. J Am Coll Cardiol 2020;76(1):122–4.

73. Wijaya I, Andhika R, Huang I. The Use of Therapeutic-Dose Anticoagulation and Its Effect on Mortality in Patients With COVID-19: A Systematic Review. Clin Appl Thromb Off J Int Acad Clin Appl Thromb 2020;26.1076029620960797.

74. Gutierrez BA, Fanola C BJ. Management of PE - American College of Cardiology. Available at: https://www.acc.org/latest-in-cardiology/articles/2020/01/27/07/42/management-of-pe. Accessed October 19, 2022.

75. Pasrija C, Kronfli A, Rouse M, et al. Outcomes after surgical pulmonary embolectomy for acute submassive and massive pulmonary embolism: A single-center experience. J Thorac Cardiovasc Surg 2018;155(3):1095–106.e2.

76. FLowTriever for Acute Massive Pulmonary Embolism (FLAME) - Full Text View - ClinicalTrials.gov. Available at: https://clinicaltrials.gov/ct2/show/NCT04795167. Accessed October 19, 2022.

77. Ain DL, Albaghdadi M, Giri J, et al. Extra-corporeal membrane oxygenation and outcomes in massive pulmonary embolism: Two eras at an urban tertiary care hospital. Vasc Med 2018;23(1):60–4.

78. Pasrija C, Shah A, George P, et al. Triage and optimization: A new paradigm in the treatment of massive pulmonary embolism. J Thorac Cardiovasc Surg 2018;156(2):672–81.

79. Geller BJ, Morrow DA, Sobieszczyk P. Percutaneous right ventricular assist device for massive pulmonary embolism. Circ Cardiovasc Interv 2012;5(6):e74–5.

80. Elder M, Blank N, Kaki A, et al. Mechanical circulatory support for acute right ventricular failure in the setting of pulmonary embolism. J Interv Cardiol 2018;31(4):518–24.

Evolving Role and Clinical Evidence in the Global Practice of Balloon Pulmonary Angioplasty

Nishant Jain, MD[a],*, Sidney Perkins, MSc[b],
Anand Reddy Maligireddy, MD[c],
Kenneth Rosenfield, MD[d]

KEYWORDS

• Chronic thromboembolic pulmonary hypertension • Chronic thromboembolic pulmonary disease
• Balloon pulmonary angioplasty • Pulmonary endarterectomy • Pulmonary hypertension

KEY POINTS

• Balloon pulmonary angioplasty (BPA) is a class I indication for inoperable or residual chronic thromboembolic pulmonary hypertension and a class IIa indication for patients with symptomatic chronic thromboembolic pulmonary disease (CTEPD) without pulmonary hypertension (PH).
• BPA safety and efficacy profiles are continuously evolving with the global adoption of the procedure.
• Recent clinical trial indicates that pre-treatment with riociguat has been associated with reduced BPA-related complications.
• Further clinical trials evaluating BPA are ongoing as there is continued interest in BPA as an expanding treatment modality for chronic thromboembolic pulmonary disease.

INTRODUCTION: CHRONIC THROMBOEMBOLIC PULMONARY HYPERTENSION

Chronic thromboembolic pulmonary hypertension (CTEPH) is classified as group IV pulmonary hypertension (PH) and is a dreaded sequelae of acute pulmonary emboli.[1] CTEPH is defined as a triad of chronic vascular occlusions with exercise limitations in the setting of pre-capillary pulmonary hypertension.[2] It is hypothesized that dysregulated vascular remodeling from defective angiogenesis, delayed fibrinolysis, and formation of fibrotic bands and webs traversing the vascular lumen results in an increase in pulmonary vascular resistance (PVR) and subsequent pulmonary hypertension.[2–4] Additionally, turbulent blood flow

and elevated pressures in the pulmonary vasculature contribute to peripheral vascular remodeling, similar to what is seen in pre-capillary PH, although this phenomenon is less understood.[5]

The incidence of CTEPH after acute pulmonary embolism (PE) ranges from 0.5 to 4.0%, contributing to 500 to 2500 annual cases in the United States alone.[6,7] Only a minority of acute PE survivors develop CTEPH and little is known as to why some patients develop CTEPH while others do not. To date, there has been no specific genetic mutation linked with the development of CTEPH.[2] Furthermore, it has been thought that CTEPH is underdiagnosed due to radiological and clinical challenges in differentiating acute from pre-existing CTEPH coupled

[a] Department of Internal Medicine, University of Michigan, Ann Arbor, MI, USA; [b] University of Michigan Medical School, Ann Arbor, MI, USA; [c] Division of Cardiology, Mayo Clinic, Scottsdale, AZ, USA; [d] Division of Cardiology, Department of Internal Medicine, Massachusetts General Hospital, Boston, MA, USA
* Corresponding author. 1500 East Medical Center Drive, Ann Arbor, MI 48109.
E-mail address: nishanja@med.umich.edu

Intervent Cardiol Clin 12 (2023) 417–427
https://doi.org/10.1016/j.iccl.2023.03.008
2211-7458/23/Published by Elsevier Inc.

with the limited access to expert CTEPH centers.[3] Regardless, CTEPH is diagnosed after 3 months of effective anticoagulation to help distinguish it from acute–subacute PE after, a right heart catheterization is required to establish a pre-capillary PH (ie, mean pulmonary artery pressure $\geq$25 mm Hg and pulmonary capillary wedge pressure $\leq$15 mm Hg).[8] Then, evidence of mismatched perfusion defects is required on ventilation-perfusion (V/Q) scan and computerized tomography (CT) angiography, MRI, or pulmonary angiography.[8] V/Q lung scan is the first line imaging modality and is 96% to 97% sensitive and 90% to 95% specific.[8] CT pulmonary angiography can augment the diagnostic yield, which may display a mosaic parenchymal pattern.[2] Additionally, CT pulmonary angiography can help identify complications of the disease, such as pulmonary artery dilation causing left main coronary artery compression, or hypertrophied bronchial arterial collaterals, which can contribute to hemoptysis.[2] Current guidelines recommend referral to an expert center for confirmation of CTEPH.[8]

Pulmonary endarterectomy (PEA) remains the treatment of choice for CTEPH and in a majority of patients who can tolerate the procedure, PEA substantially improves hemodynamics and long-term mortality (ie, 89% vs 70% 3-year survival in operated vs non-operated, respectively).[9] However, PEA for CTEPH may necessitate bilateral PEA, which often requires extracorporeal membrane oxygenation support, and has a reported ~5% in-hospital mortality.[9] Surgical candidacy varies from center to center, and in a large multi-national registry analysis of 1010 patients, only 669 patients (66%) were considered operable candidates and of these candidates, only 593 patients (59%) received PEA.[10] Thus, there is a substantial population with inoperable or inaccessible CTEPH. Current guidelines now recommend balloon pulmonary angioplasty (BPA), a non-surgical interventional treatment, for patients with inoperable or inaccessible CTEPH; in this review, we hope to highlight the evolution of BPA in the treatment of CTEPH (Fig. 1).

EARLY ERA OF BALLOON PULMONARY ANGIOPLASTY (2001 TO 2018)

Before 2001, the mainstay treatment of inoperable CTEPH was anticoagulation alone.[11] In 2001, Feinstein and colleagues published a landmark case series of 18 patients introducing BPA as an interventional option that can successfully improve New York Heart Association (NYHA) class, 6-minute walking distances, and mean pulmonary artery pressures for patients with inaccessible CTEPH.[11] However in this small cohort, 11 patients developed reperfusion edema and three required mechanical ventilation.[11]

After 2001, BPA evolved initially in Japan, where the procedure was refined in large patient cohorts across PH centers, using smaller balloons and limiting the number of balloon inflations.[12] These refinements were evaluated for efficacy and complications with imaging (CT, echocardiogram, MRI), invasive hemodynamics, and cardiopulmonary exercise testing.[12–15] With refinement in technique and large-scale implementation, BPA expanded globally in PH centers worldwide, including Germany, United States, France, the Netherlands, United Kingdom, China, and many more (Table 1).

In 2015, the European Society of Cardiology (ESC) and the European Respiratory Society (ERS) gave a class IIb recommendation that interventional BPA may be considered in patients who are technically non-operable or carry an unfavorable risk–benefit ratio for PEA.[2] Before these recommendations, CHEST-1 and CHEST-2 trials were published demonstrating that riociguat, a soluble guanylate cyclase stimulator, improved exercise capacity and PVR, with favorable 1-year follow-up, and so, in 2015, ESC/ERS guidelines granted a class Ib recommendation for the use of riociguat, the only FDA-approved CTEPH pulmonary vasodilator medication, for persistent/recurrent or inoperable CTEPH.[2,16–18]

In 2017, a Polish center compared BPA, PEA, and medical therapy alone with long-term, ie, 3- to 5-year follow-up and found BPA to have a higher cumulative survival rate when compared to PEA (P =.39) and medical therapy (P =.02).[19] In this study, they described a refined, less aggressive BPA strategy including, avoidance of total, subtotal occlusions, pouch lesions, use of smaller, undersized balloon catheters, and less aggressive anticoagulation.[19] In 2018, updated recommendations from the Cologne Consensus Conference found BPA to be increasingly prevalent across European countries, suggesting a shift in practice patterns and a need for updated recommendations.[20]

CURRENT PRACTICE OF BALLOON PULMONARY ANGIOPLASTY (2018 TO PRESENT)

Since the 2018 Cologne Consensus Conference, there has been a large explosion of BPA

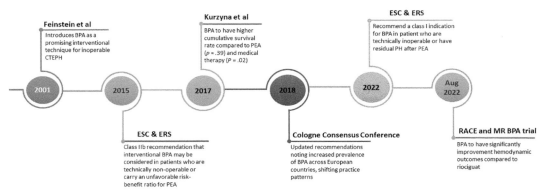

Fig. 1. Balloon Pulmonary Angioplasty: Inception to present. timeline of balloon pulmonary angioplasty milestones.

procedures across PH centers worldwide. The current practice of BPA involves the use of intravascular ultrasound (IVUS), pressure-guided wires, and advanced imaging to optimize lesion selection and reduce complication rates with BPA.[12,21,22] Reports out of Japan suggest preferentially targeting ring-like and web lesions, with consideration of avoiding total occlusion/pouch lesions or tortuous lesions to reduce complications.[21,22] The use of pressure wire can be used to help reduce complications. Brisk return of blood flow, or grade 3 pulmonary flow, is thought to be the gold standard, but some reports indicate that a pressure ratio of greater than 0.8 can also be useful in indicating sufficient dilation.[22] Furthermore, pressure distal to the lesion should not exceed 35 mm Hg to avoid reperfusion pulmonary edema.[23] IVUS and optical frequency domain imaging (OFDI) have been applied to BPA with safe, feasible, and favorable results, albeit in small case series, and further studies are needed.[12] A limited case series (n = 9) showed interval benefit to optical coherence tomography (OCT) compared to IVUS in terms of chronic thromboembolus detection, although complication rates were not assessed.[24] BPA has been performed with evidence of radiographic benefit on imaging modalities, including ECHO, MRI, and CT, and some case series have also noted improvement in quality of life after BPA.[14,15,25]

Efficacy Outcomes

In a large, single-center French study, BPA performed for inoperable CTEPH was described between initial and recent periods (split date: March 2017).[26] In this study, efficacy outcomes showed a reduction in mPAP and PVR in initial versus recent periods (22% versus 37% [P

=.001], 38% versus 53% [P =.002], respectively).[26] Improvements in the recent period were attributed to the significant learning curve with BPA.[26] Similar improvements in hemodynamic parameters have been seen in a large multi-center Polish registry containing 236 patients who underwent 1056 BPA procedures (mPAP reduced by 14.9 mm Hg [P<.001], PVR reduced by 4.0 WU [P<.001], and 6 MWT increased by 82 m [P<.001]).[27] Centers across the globe have noted improvement in hemodynamic parameters, including a multi-center Japanese center,[28] a large Chinese center,[29] a large UK center,[15] and others.

Safety Outcomes

In terms of safety, BPA-related complications have remained at the forefront of discussion in regards to hesitation in adoption of BPA as reports from Feinstein and colleagues noted significant rates of hemoptysis, reperfusion edema, mechanical ventilation, and mortality.[11] With refinement in the BPA technique, the safety profile has evolved, primarily from smaller balloon size and less aggressive anticoagulation strategies, given the fragility of the pulmonary vasculature.[19,26] A pooled cohort analysis comparing BPA-related complications from 18 countries (n=1,714 patients) found from the first period (2013-2017) to the second period (2018-2022), the cumulative incidence of hemoptysis/vascular injury decreased from 14.1% to 7.7% (P<.01); lung injury/reperfusion edema decreased from 11.3% to 1.4% (P<.01); invasive mechanical ventilation decreased from 0.7% to 0.1% (P<.01); and mortality decreased from 2.0% to 0.8% (P<.01).[30] The improvement in periprocedural complications was attributed to refined patient selection and procedural technique.[30]

Table 1
Summary of literature

Location	First Author Year	BPA Sessions	Patients	Follow-up, in months	NYHA	6MWD	BNP	QoL	Pulmonary Hemo-dynamics	ECHO	CT	MRI	CPET	Complications
Boston—USA	Feinstein et al,[11] 2001	1994–1999	47	18	36	✓	✓			✓					✓
Oslo—Norway	Broch et al,[33] 2016	2003–2014	NR	32	35	✓	✓	✓		✓	✓				
Prague—Czech Republic	Jansa et al,[34] 2020	2003–2019	160	64	3	✓	✓	✓	✓	✓					✓
Okayama—Japan	Mizoguchi et al,[12] 2012	2004–2011	255	68	26	✓	✓	✓	✓	✓					✓
Tokyo—Japan	Inami et al,[13] 2014	2009–2013	213	68	3	✓	✓	✓		✓					✓
	Inami et al,[23] 2014	2009–2013	350	103	14	✓	✓	✓		✓	✓				✓
	Moriyama et al,[35] 2018	2011–2016	318	53	NR	✓	✓	✓		✓					
	Tsugu et al,[36] 2015	2012–2014	NR	25	NR	✓	✓	✓		✓	✓				
	Tsukada et al,[37] 2021	2012–2016	525	82	6	✓	✓	✓		✓			✓		
	Nishiyama et al,[38] 2018	2017	360	60	6	✓	✓	✓		✓	✓				

Center	Study	Period			
Tohuko—Japan	Aoki et al,[25] 2017	2009–2016	424	84	42
	Akizuki et al,[39] 2017	2012–2014	62	13	3
Osaka—Japan	Ogo et al,[40] 2017	2011–2015	385	80	12
Kobe—Japan	Taniguchi et al,[41] 2021	2011–2019	324	81	2.7
Suita—Japan	Fukui et al,[42] 2014	2012–2013	64	20	4
Nagasaki—Japan	Yamagata et al,[43] 2018	2013–2016	31	11	1
Madrid—Spain	Velazquez et al,[44] 2019	2013–2017	156	46	15.3
Kyushu—Japan	Yamazaki et al,[45] 2017	2013–2017	102	29	16.8
Hanover—Germany	Maschke et al,[46] 2019	2013–2017	266	67	1
	Schoenfeld et al,[14] 2019	2014–2016	NR	29	2
Bad Nauheim—Germany	Wiedenroth et al,[47] 2020	2014–2018	358	64	6
Leuven—Belgium		2014–2018	91	18	1

(continued on next page)

Table 1
(*continued*)

Location	First Author	Year	BPA Sessions	Patients	Follow-up, in months	NYHA	6MWD	BNP	QoL	Pulmonary Hemo-dynamics	ECHO	CT	MRI	CPET	Complications
	Godinas et al,[48] 2019														
Paris—France	Brenot et al,[49] 2019	2014–2017	1006	184	6.1	✔	✔			✔					✔
Warsaw—Poland	Roik et al,[50] 2016	2014–2015	27	9	5	✔	✔	✔							✔
Rochester— USA	Anand et al,[51] 2019	2014–2018	75	31	NR	✔	✔			✔	✔				✔
Taiwan	Chen et al,[52] 2021	2014–2020	59	13	21	✔	✔	✔		✔	✔				✔
Amsterdam — The Netherlands	van Thor et al,[53] 2020	2015–2019	172	38	6	✔	✔	✔		✔					✔
Seoul— Korea	Kwon et al,[54] 2018	2015–2017	52	15	6	✔	✔			✔	✔				✔
Krakow— Poland	Magon et al,[55] 2019	2015–2017	103	17	6	✔	✔	✔		✔					
UK	Hoole et al,[15] 2020	2015–2018	95	30	3	✔	✔	✔	✔	✔	✔			✔	✔
Beijing—China	Zhang et al,[56] 2020	2016–2019	137	46	0						✔				

Center	Reference	Years											
Chile	Sepulveda et al,[57] 2021	2016–2019	81	22	17.3	✓	✓	✓	✓			✓	
Otwock—Poland	Kurzyna et al,[19] 2017	2017	157	56	24	✓	✓	✓	✓			✓	
Israel	Segel et al,[58] 2020	2017	47	5	5 to 11	✓	✓	✓	✓			✓	
Paris—France	Jais et al,[32] 2022	2016–2019	400	52	12	✓	✓	✓	✓			✓	
Multi-Center Japan	Kawakami et al,[28] 2022	2016–2019	150	32	12	✓	✓	✓	✓			✓	
Almada—Portugal	Cale et al[59]	2017–2019	57	11	6	✓	✓	✓	✓			✓	
Beijing—China	Jin et al,[60] 2019	2018–2019	40	25	0	✓	✓	✓	✓	✓	✓	✓	✓
Istanbul—Turkey	Kanar et al,[61] 2019	2019	52	20	3	✓	✓	✓			✓		
Grenoble—France	Piliero et al,[26] 2022	2013–2020	646	156	6	✓	✓	✓	✓			✓	
Guangzhou—China	Hong et al,[29] 2022	2019–2021	210	92	0	✓	✓		✓			✓	
San Diego—USA	Mahmud et al,[62] 2021	2021	164	39	NR	✓	✓	✓	✓			✓	

Summary of Global PH center data since 2001 including English-printed manuscripts and clinical trials and excluding case reports, case series (less than five patients), abstracts, and review articles.

Current Guidelines

Now, given the evolving and improving nature of BPA in the current era and the large global adoption of BPA, 2022 ESC/ERS guidelines recommend a class I indication for "BPA in patients who are technically inoperable or have residual PH after PEA and distal obstructions amenable to BPA."[8] Additionally, there is an IIa recommendation for BPA to be considered in patients with symptomatic CTEPD without PH.[8] The latter recommendation stems from a small case series from Germany, in which patients with inoperable CTEPD without PH benefited from BPA.[31]

Recent Clinical Trials

Furthermore, two major clinical trials have been published simultaneously since these recommendations evaluating the role of riociguat versus BPA in inoperable CTEPH. The RACE trial in France is a multi-center, phase 3, open-labeled, randomized controlled trial and found BPA to have a more pronounced reduction in PVR compared to riociguat.[32] More treatment-related serious adverse events were seen in the BPA arm, but interestingly, fewer serious adverse events were observed if patients were pre-treated with riociguat, highlighting a potential role for multimodal, sequential treatment protocols.[32] The MR BPA trial in Japan was also a multi-center, open-labeled, randomized controlled trial and similarly found BPA to be associated with a greater reduction in mPAP, however with increased procedure-related complications.[28]

FUTURE DIRECTIONS

Further clinical trials evaluating BPA are ongoing as there is continued interest in BPA as an expanding treatment modality for CTEPD. Still, there lacks of standardization of BPA procedure and endpoints across PH centers, which complicates outcomes research and registry design. Several ongoing trials are examining the utility of exercise rehab (EXPECT-PH Trial, University of Michigan, Ann Arbor, MI; CPETPH Trial, Fuwai Hospital, Beijing, China; and POpPART Trial, University Hospital, Grenoble, France); adjuvant medications such as riociguat and macitentan (THERAPY-HYBRID-BPA, Okayama Medical Center, Japan; IMPACT-CTEPH, Hôpital de Paris, Paris, France; EPIPHANY, Duke University, Durham, NC); and safety and efficacy of BPA compared head-to-head with PEA (GO-CTEPH, University of Aarhus, Vienna, Austria). Long-term clinical success and safety data are needed

for the advancement of BPA. More guidance is also needed for optimal patient selection for BPA as it continues to expand in centers worldwide.

CLINICS CARE POINTS

- Balloon pulmonary angioplasty (BPA) is a class I indication for inoperable or residual chronic thromboembolic pulmonary hypertension and a class IIa indication for patients with symptomatic CTEPD without PH.
- With refinement in the BPA technique, the safety profile has evolved, primarily from smaller balloon size and less aggressive anticoagulation strategies, given the fragility of the pulmonary vasculature.
- Recent clinical trials suggest pretreatment with riociguat may lower BPA complications.

DISCLOSURE

Dr K. Rosenfield holds equity and reports serving on advisory boards for Althea Medical. Dr K. Rosenfield reports serving as a consultant for Angiodynamics, Boston Scientific, Contego Medical, Neptune Medical, Penumbra, Philips. Dr K. Rosenfield is a principal investigator or co-investigator on research grants from the NIH, United States, and Boston Scientific, United States. All other authors have no relevant relationships to disclose.

REFERENCES

1. Lang I. Chronic thromboembolic pulmonary hypertension: a distinct disease entity. Eur Respir Rev 2015;24(136):246–52.
2. Galiè N, Humbert M, Vachiery JL, et al. 2015 ESC/ERS Guidelines for the diagnosis and treatment of pulmonary hypertension: The Joint Task Force for the Diagnosis and Treatment of Pulmonary Hypertension of the European Society of Cardiology (ESC) and the European Respiratory Society (ERS): Endorsed by: Association for European Paediatric and Congenital Cardiology (AEPC), International Society for Heart and Lung Transplantation (ISHLT). Eur Heart J 2016;37(1):67–119.
3. Galiè N, Hoeper MM, Humbert M, et al. Guidelines for the diagnosis and treatment of pulmonary hypertension: the Task Force for the Diagnosis and Treatment of Pulmonary Hypertension of the

European Society of Cardiology (ESC) and the European Respiratory Society (ERS), endorsed by the International Society of Heart and Lung Transplantation (ISHLT). Eur Heart J 2009;30(20):2493–537.

4. Fedullo PF, Auger WR, Kerr KM, et al. Chronic thromboembolic pulmonary hypertension. N Engl J Med 2001;345(20):1465–72.

5. Logue R, Safdar Z. Chronic Thromboembolic Pulmonary Hypertension Medical Management. Methodi DeBak Cardiovasc J 2021;17(2):e29.

6. Tapson VF, Humbert M. Incidence and Prevalence of Chronic Thromboembolic Pulmonary Hypertension. Proc Am Thorac Soc 2006;3(7):564–7.

7. Delcroix M, Kerr K, Fedullo P. Chronic Thromboembolic Pulmonary Hypertension. Epidemiology and Risk Factors. Ann Am Thorac Soc 2016; 13(Supplement_3):S201–6.

8. Humbert M, Kovacs G, Hoeper MM, et al. 2022 ESC/ERS Guidelines for the diagnosis and treatment of pulmonary hypertension: Developed by the task force for the diagnosis and treatment of pulmonary hypertension of the European Society of Cardiology (ESC) and the European Respiratory Society (ERS). Endorsed by the International Society for Heart and Lung Transplantation (ISHLT) and the European Reference Network on rare respiratory diseases (ERN-LUNG). Eur Heart J 2022;ehac237.

9. Delcroix M, Lang I, Pepke-Zaba J, et al. Long-Term Outcome of Patients With Chronic Thromboembolic Pulmonary Hypertension: Results From an International Prospective Registry. Circulation 2016; 133(9):859–71.

10. Guth S, D'Armini AM, Delcroix M, et al. Current strategies for managing chronic thromboembolic pulmonary hypertension: results of the worldwide prospective CTEPH Registry. ERJ Open Res 2021; 7(3).

11. Feinstein JA, Goldhaber SZ, Lock JE, et al. Balloon pulmonary angioplasty for treatment of chronic thromboembolic pulmonary hypertension. Circulation 2001;103(1):10–3.

12. Mizoguchi H, Ogawa A, Munemasa M, et al. Refined Balloon Pulmonary Angioplasty for Inoperable Patients with Chronic Thromboembolic Pulmonary Hypertension. Circ Cardiovasc Interv 2012;5(6):748–55.

13. Inami T, Kataoka M, Ando M, et al. A New Era of Therapeutic Strategies for Chronic Thromboembolic Pulmonary Hypertension by Two Different Interventional Therapies; Pulmonary Endarterectomy and Percutaneous Transluminal Pulmonary Angioplasty. PLoS One 2014;9(4):e94587.

14. Schoenfeld C, Hinrichs JB, Olsson KM, et al. Cardio-pulmonary MRI for detection of treatment response after a single BPA treatment session in CTEPH patients. Eur Radiol 2019;29(4):1693–702.

15. Hoole SP, Coghlan JG, Cannon JE, et al. Balloon pulmonary angioplasty for inoperable chronic thromboembolic pulmonary hypertension: the UK experience. Open Heart 2020;7(1):e001144.

16. Ghofrani H-A, D'Armini AM, Grimminger F, et al. Riociguat for the Treatment of Chronic Thromboembolic Pulmonary Hypertension. N Engl J Med 2013;369(4):319–29.

17. Donaldson S, Ogunti R, Kibreab A, et al. Riociguat in the Treatment of Chronic Thromboembolic Pulmonary Hypertension: An Evidence-Based Review of Its Place in Therapy. Core Evid 2020;15:31–40.

18. Simonneau G, D'Armini AM, Ghofrani HA, et al. Riociguat for the treatment of chronic thromboembolic pulmonary hypertension: a long-term extension study (CHEST-2). Eur Respir J 2015;45(5): 1293–302.

19. Kurzyna M, Darocha S, Pietura R, et al. Changing the strategy of balloon pulmonary angioplasty resulted in a reduced complication rate in patients with chronic thromboembolic pulmonary hypertension. A single-centre European experience. Kardiol Pol 2017;75(7):645–54.

20. Wilkens H, Konstantinides S, Lang IM, et al. Chronic thromboembolic pulmonary hypertension (CTEPH): Updated Recommendations from the Cologne Consensus Conference 2018. Int J Cardiol 2018; 272s:69–78.

21. Kawakami T, Ogawa A, Miyaji K, et al. Novel Angiographic Classification of Each Vascular Lesion in Chronic Thromboembolic Pulmonary Hypertension Based on Selective Angiogram and Results of Balloon Pulmonary Angioplasty. Circ Cardiovasc Interv 2016;9(10):e003318.

22. Kataoka M, Inami T, Kawakami T, et al. Balloon Pulmonary Angioplasty (Percutaneous Transluminal Pulmonary Angioplasty) for Chronic Thromboembolic Pulmonary Hypertension: A Japanese Perspective. JACC Cardiovasc Interv 2019;12(14): 1382–8.

23. Inami T, Kataoka M, Shimura N, et al. Pressure-wire-guided percutaneous transluminal pulmonary angioplasty: a breakthrough in catheter-interventional therapy for chronic thromboembolic pulmonary hypertension. JACC Cardiovasc Interv 2014;7(11): 1297–306.

24. Tatebe S, Fukumoto Y, Sugimura K, et al. Optical Coherence Tomography Is Superior to Intravascular Ultrasound for Diagnosis of Distal-Type Chronic Thromboembolic Pulmonary Hypertension. Circ J 2013;77(4):1081–3.

25. Aoki T, Sugimura K, Tatebe S, et al. Comprehensive evaluation of the effectiveness and safety of balloon pulmonary angioplasty for inoperable chronic thrombo-embolic pulmonary hypertension: long-term effects and procedure-related complications. Eur Heart J 2017;38(42):3152–9.

26. Piliero N, Thony F, Guillien A, et al. Balloon pulmonary angioplasty for chronic thromboembolic pulmonary hypertension: Evaluation of haemodynamic effects, complication rates and radiation exposure over time. Arch Cardiovasc Dis 2022;115(5):295–304.

27. Szymon D, Marek R, Grzegorz K, et al. Balloon pulmonary angioplasty in chronic thromboembolic pulmonary hypertension: a multicentre registry. EuroIntervention 2022;17(13):1104–11.

28. Kawakami T, Matsubara H, Shinke T, et al. Balloon pulmonary angioplasty versus riociguat in inoperable chronic thromboembolic pulmonary hypertension (MR BPA): an open-label, randomised controlled trial. Lancet Respir Med 2022;10(10):949–60.

29. Hong C, Lu J, Wu X, et al. Bilateral versus unilateral balloon pulmonary angioplasty for inoperable chronic thromboembolic pulmonary hypertension. Respir Res 2022;23(1):117.

30. Jain N, Sheikh MA, Bajaj D, et al. Periprocedural Complications With Balloon Pulmonary Angioplasty: Analysis of Global Studies. JACC: Cardiovascular Interventions 2023.

31. Wiedenroth CB, Olsson KM, Guth S, et al. Balloon pulmonary angioplasty for inoperable patients with chronic thromboembolic disease. Pulm Circ 2017; 8(1). 2045893217753122.

32. Jaïs X, Brenot P, Bouvaist H, et al. Balloon pulmonary angioplasty versus riociguat for the treatment of inoperable chronic thromboembolic pulmonary hypertension (RACE): a multicentre, phase 3, open-label, randomised controlled trial and ancillary follow-up study. Lancet Respir Med 2022; 10(10):961–71.

33. Broch K, Murbraech K, Ragnarsson A, et al. Echocardiographic evidence of right ventricular functional improvement after balloon pulmonary angioplasty in chronic thromboembolic pulmonary hypertension. J Heart Lung Transplant 2016;35(1): 80–6.

34. Jansa P, Heller S, Svoboda M, et al. Balloon Pulmonary Angioplasty in Patients with Chronic Thromboembolic Pulmonary Hypertension: Impact on Clinical and Hemodynamic Parameters, Quality of Life and Risk Profile. J Clin Med 2020;9(11):3608.

35. Moriyama H, Murata M, Tsugu T, et al. The clinical value of assessing right ventricular diastolic function after balloon pulmonary angioplasty in patients with chronic thromboembolic pulmonary hypertension. Int J Cardiovasc Imag 2018;34(6): 875–82.

36. Tsugu T, Murata M, Kawakami T, et al. Significance of Echocardiographic Assessment for Right Ventricular Function After Balloon Pulmonary Angioplasty in Patients With Chronic Thromboembolic Induced Pulmonary Hypertension. Am J Cardiol 2015;115(2): 256–61.

37. Tsukada J, Yamada Y, Kawakami T, et al. Treatment effect prediction using CT after balloon pulmonary angioplasty in chronic thromboembolic pulmonary hypertension. Eur Radiol 2021;31(8):5524–32.

38. Nishiyama T, Takatsuki S, Kawakami T, et al. Improvement in the electrocardiograms associated with right ventricular hypertrophy after balloon pulmonary angioplasty in chronic thromboembolic pulmonary hypertension. Int J Cardiol Heart Vasc 2018;19:75–82.

39. Akizuki M, Serizawa N, Ueno A, et al. Effect of Balloon Pulmonary Angioplasty on Respiratory Function in Patients With Chronic Thromboembolic Pulmonary Hypertension. Chest 2017;151(3):643–9.

40. Ogo T, Fukuda T, Tsuji A, et al. Efficacy and safety of balloon pulmonary angioplasty for chronic thromboembolic pulmonary hypertension guided by cone-beam computed tomography and electrocardiogram-gated area detector computed tomography. Eur J Radiol 2017;89:270–6.

41. Taniguchi Y, Matsuoka Y, Onishi H, et al. The role of balloon pulmonary angioplasty and pulmonary endarterectomy: Is chronic thromboembolic pulmonary hypertension still a life-threatening disease? Int J Cardiol 2021;326:170–7.

42. Fukui S, Ogo T, Morita Y, et al. Right ventricular reverse remodelling after balloon pulmonary angioplasty. Eur Respir J 2014;43(5):1394–402.

43. Yamagata Y, Ikeda S, Nakata T, et al. Balloon pulmonary angioplasty is effective for treating peripheral-type chronic thromboembolic pulmonary hypertension in elderly patients. Geriatr Gerontol Int 2018;18(5):678–84.

44. Velázquez M, Albarrán A, Hernández I, et al. Balloon Pulmonary Angioplasty for Inoperable Patients With Chronic Thromboembolic Pulmonary Hypertension. Observational Study in a Referral Unit. Rev Esp Cardiol 2019;72(3):224–32.

45. Yamasaki Y, Nagao M, Abe K, et al. Balloon pulmonary angioplasty improves interventricular dyssynchrony in patients with inoperable chronic thromboembolic pulmonary hypertension: a cardiac MR imaging study. Int J Cardiovasc Imaging 2017;33(2):229–39.

46. Maschke SK, Hinrichs JB, Renne J, et al. C-Arm computed tomography (CACT)-guided balloon pulmonary angioplasty (BPA): Evaluation of patient safety and peri- and post-procedural complications. Eur Radiol 2019;29(3):1276–84.

47. Wiedenroth CB, Rieth AJ, Kriechbaum S, et al. Exercise right heart catheterization before and after balloon pulmonary angioplasty in inoperable patients with chronic thromboembolic pulmonary hypertension. Pulm Circ 2020;10(3). 2045894020917884.

48. Godinas L, Bonne L, Budts W, et al. Balloon Pulmonary Angioplasty for the Treatment of Nonoperable Chronic Thromboembolic Pulmonary Hypertension:

Single-Center Experience with Low Initial Complication Rate. J Vasc Interv Radiol 2019;30(8):1265–72.

49. Brenot P, Jaïs X, Taniguchi Y, et al. French experience of balloon pulmonary angioplasty for chronic thromboembolic pulmonary hypertension. Eur Respir J 2019;53(5):1802095.

50. Roik M, Wretowski D, Łabyk A, et al. Refined balloon pulmonary angioplasty driven by combined assessment of intra-arterial anatomy and physiology – Multimodal approach to treated lesions in patients with non-operable distal chronic thromboembolic pulmonary hypertension – Technique, safety and efficacy of 50 consecutive angioplasties. Int J Cardiol 2016;203:228–35.

51. Anand V, Frantz RP, DuBrock H, et al. Balloon Pulmonary Angioplasty for Chronic Thromboembolic Pulmonary Hypertension: Initial Single-Center Experience. Mayo Clin Proc Innov Qual Outcomes 2019;3(3):311–8.

52. Chen ZW, Wu CK, Kuo PH, et al. Efficacy and safety of balloon pulmonary angioplasty in patients with inoperable chronic thromboembolic pulmonary hypertension. J Formos Med Assoc 2021;120(3):947–55.

53. van Thor MCJ, Lely RJ, Braams NJ, et al. Safety and efficacy of balloon pulmonary angioplasty in chronic thromboembolic pulmonary hypertension in the Netherlands. Neth Heart J 2020;28(2):81–8.

54. Kwon W, Yang JH, Park TK, et al. Impact of Balloon Pulmonary Angioplasty on Hemodynamics and Clinical Outcomes in Patients with Chronic Thromboembolic Pulmonary Hypertension: the Initial Korean Experience. J Korean Med Sci 2018;33(4):e24.

55. Magoń W, Stępniewski J, Waligóra M, et al. Pulmonary Artery Elastic Properties After Balloon Pulmonary Angioplasty in Patients With Inoperable Chronic Thromboembolic Pulmonary Hypertension. Can J Cardiol 2019;35(4):422–9.

56. Zhang X, Guo D, Wang J, et al. Speckle tracking for predicting outcomes of balloon pulmonary angioplasty in patients with chronic thromboembolic pulmonary hypertension. Echocardiography 2020;37(6):841–9.

57. Sepúlveda P, Hameau R, Backhouse C, et al. Midterm follow-up of balloon pulmonary angioplasty for inoperable chronic thromboembolic pulmonary hypertension: An experience in Latin America. Catheter Cardiovasc Interv 2021;97(6):E748–57.

58. Segel MJ, Somech D, Lang IM, et al. Balloon Pulmonary Angioplasty for Inoperable Chronic Thromboembolic Pulmonary Hypertension: First Experience at the Israeli National CTEPH Referral Center. Isr Med Assoc J 2020;22(12):752–6.

59. Calé R, Ferreira F, Pereira AR, et al. Safety and efficacy of balloon pulmonary angioplasty in a Portuguese pulmonary hypertension expert center. Revista portuguesa de cardiologia (English ed) 2021;40(10):727–37.

60. Jin Q, Luo Q, Yang T, et al. Improved hemodynamics and cardiopulmonary function in patients with inoperable chronic thromboembolic pulmonary hypertension after balloon pulmonary angioplasty. Respir Res 2019;20(1):250.

61. Kanar BG, Mutlu B, Atas H, et al. Improvements of right ventricular function and hemodynamics after balloon pulmonary angioplasty in patients with chronic thromboembolic pulmonary hypertension. Echocardiography 2019;36(11):2050–6.

62. Mahmud E, Patel M, Ang L, et al. Advances in balloon pulmonary angioplasty for chronic thromboembolic pulmonary hypertension. Pulm Circ 2021;11(2). 20458940211007385.

Outpatient Follow-up of Pulmonary Embolism
Putting It all Together

Muhammad Adil Sheikh, MD[a],*,
Gabriella VanAken, MD candidate[b],
Syed Nabeel Hyder, MD[c], Jay Giri, MD[d]

KEYWORDS

- Pulmonary embolism • Chronic thromboembolic disease
- Chronic thromboembolic pulmonary hypertension • Post-PE syndrome
- Pulmonary embolism response team

KEY POINTS

- Focused and coordinated care is required for long-term management of pulmonary embolism.
- Anticoagulants, complications of PE such as manifestations of the Post-PE syndrome, thrombophilia testing and IVC filters are key areas to address in outpatient follow-up.
- A dedicated long-term outpatient follow-up clinic streamlines this care to potentially avoid complications and improve patients' quality of life.

INTRODUCTION

Pulmonary embolism (PE) is a leading cause of cardiovascular morbidity and mortality worldwide.[1] It accounts for approximately 100,000 deaths annually in the United States and is directly related to 5% to 10% of all in-hospital deaths.[2] Although inpatient mortality with PE continues to be a significant concern, recent data have also suggested about 30% of all PE survivors die within the first year of discharge.[3]

The natural history of PE typically includes restoration of normal hemodynamics and gas exchange and full resolution of thromboemboli or minimal residual thrombosis within 30 days.[4] Although PE was once regarded as a disease whereby full recovery was expected with anticoagulation, it has now been learned that PE can lead to several complications despite adequate anticoagulation.[5] These complications include an increased risk for recurrent deep venous thrombosis (DVT) and PE, bleeding from anticoagulant therapy, chronic thromboembolic disease (CTED) with and without associated pulmonary arterial hypertension (PAH), and the more recently described other phenotypes of post-PE syndrome.[6–12]

More than one-third of all patients discharged after an acute PE were found to have inconsistent follow-up, and insufficient workup for chronic complications of PE despite reporting persistent symptoms. There was also a wide variation in how follow-up testing was performed with no relation to signs and symptoms.[13] The authors' experience with PE response teams (PERT) in the inpatient setting has demonstrated that having a dedicated multidisciplinary service for patients with PE can be very useful in enhancing care quality. This same model can also be extended to the outpatient setting, where a dedicated multidisciplinary PE clinic can bring expertise from various disciplines together, enhancing overall patient care.

[a] Division of Cardiology, Department of Internal Medicine, Southern Illinois University, PO Box 19636, Springfield, IL 62794-9636, USA; [b] University of Michigan School of Medicine, 1500 East Medical Center Drive, Ann Arbor, MI 48109, USA; [c] Division of Cardiology, Department of Internal Medicine, University of Michigan, 1500 East Medical Center Drive, Ann Arbor, MI 48109, USA; [d] Cardiovascular Medicine Division, Department of Medicine, Hospital of the University of Pennsylvania, 3400 Civic Center Boulevard, Philadelphia, PA 19104, USA
* Corresponding author.
E-mail addresses: madilsheikh@gmail.com; msheikh44@siumed.edu

The authors believe that a dedicated PE follow-up clinic extends the organized, systematic care provided to inpatient patients with PE via the PERT model in the outpatient setting. Such an initiative may standardizes follow-up protocols after PE, limits unnecessary tests, while ensuring adequate management of those who develop chronic complications such as CTED, CTEPH, and the lesser-defined phenotypes of post-PE syndrome.

PROPOSED FRAMEWORK FOR A PULMONARY EMBOLISM CLINIC

A PE clinic's fundamental purpose is to systematically screen and work up those with persistent functional decline using careful history taking, standardized questionnaires, and other imaging studies. Other important issues addressed include assessing the underlying risk factors for PE (provoked vs unprovoked), thrombophilia evaluation, occult malignancy screening, management of anticoagulation, and assessing the continued need for inferior vena cava (IVC) filter if placed during the index PE episode.[14]

Assessment of Functional Status
A comprehensive assessment of functional status post-PE is critical in follow-up. Patients who remain limited and symptomatic after 3 months of anticoagulant treatment should be assessed for CTED and are those who benefit most from the dedicated multidisciplinary care.

The Pulmonary Embolism Quality of Life (PEmb-QoL, Appendix 1) questionnaire, developed in 2009,[15] and the post–venous thromboembolism (VTE) functional status (PVFS, Appendix 2) scale, initially developed in 2019 and further modified in 2020,[16] are disease-specific tools useful for assessing quality of life and functional status, respectively, after an acute PE. The general health-related quality-of-life questionnaire short form–36[17] is another option, but PEmb-QoL and PVFS are disease-specific and are preferred. These tools serve as adjuncts to a careful history and physical examination. They are particularly useful in objectively quantifying and tracking patients with post-PE syndrome on longitudinal follow-up.

Postpulmonary embolism syndrome and its clinical phenotypes
After an acute PE, persistent symptomatic patients who have completed 3 months of anticoagulation fall under the umbrella of "post-PE syndrome." This syndrome encompasses persistent dyspnea, exercise limitation, and impaired quality of life beyond 3 months after an acute PE. An established description for post-PE syndrome has not been finalized thus far. Broadly, it includes patients with CTED and CTEPH (Fig. 1, adapted from Klok and colleagues).[18] The authors believe patients with PE who have persistent symptoms despite adequate anticoagulation have 3 distinct phenotypes.

1. Patients with residual thromboembolic pulmonary disease who have pulmonary hypertension (PH) with or without persistent right ventricular (RV) dysfunction (CTEPH).
2. Patients with residual thromboembolic disease without PH or persistent RV dysfunction (CTED).
3. Patients with persistent symptoms and functional limitations without residual thromboembolic disease, RV dysfunction, or PH. This group of patients with mostly unexplained dyspnea is the other not well-understood clinical phenotype of post-PE syndrome.

Fig. 2 summarizes the authors' proposed approach for diagnostic evaluation of patients with persistent dyspnea and functional limitations after 3 months of treatment of PE.

Chronic thromboembolic pulmonary hypertension
These patients have evidence of PH (at rest or with exercise) with or without residual RV dysfunction noted on follow-up (>3 months after the acute PE episode).[14,19] The ventilation-perfusion (V/Q) scan will show mismatched perfusion defects.[20–22] A normal V/Q scan essentially rules out CTEPH with a sensitivity of 90% to 100% and a specificity of 94% to 100%. Classically, V/Q scan findings in CTEPH include more than one segmental or larger mismatched perfusion defects.[22] V/Q scan findings need to be confirmed with an invasive pulmonary angiogram or cardiac tomographic pulmonary angiogram (CT-PE) to establish a CTEPH diagnosis. In contrast, a normal V/Q scan or unmatched/nonsegmental distal perfusion abnormalities secondary to diffuse narrowing of small vessels are generally seen in PH from other causes (such as PAH or pulmonary veno-occlusive disease).[23,24] An emerging alternative imaging study is dual-energy CT-PE that combines features of standard CT-PE with V/Q scanning in one study. All patients with CTEPH require life-long anticoagulation. Pulmonary thromboendarterectomy (PTE) for surgical candidates is potentially curative and is considered first-line treatment. Medical therapy and balloon pulmonary angioplasty may improve hemodynamics and symptoms in patients who are not surgical candidates due to anatomical or comborbid considerations or have persistent PH after PTE.[25]

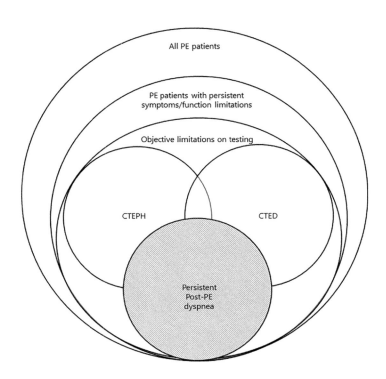

Fig. 1. Chronic complications of PE and phenotypes of post-PE syndrome.

Chronic thromboembolic pulmonary disease
Patients with V/Q scan imaging defects, but without resting PH or RV dysfunction are classified into the CTED phenotype.[20] Classically, CTED is a precursor to CTEPH, and cardiopulmonary exercise testing (CPET)[26] is often used to objectively quantify functional limitations and link increased dead space ventilation or subclinical RV dysfunction to these patients' symptoms.

Among other indices, CPET reports the maximal volume of oxygen consumption (vo_2) and carbon dioxide output (vco_2), minute ventilation, and maximum voluntary ventilation.[27] CPET findings typical of CTED include the following: reduced exercise capacity (peak oxygen consumption [peak vo_2]), increased dead space ventilation, inadequate ventilation (increased minute ventilation/carbon dioxide production slope), and a reduced O_2 pulse that may indicated reduced stroke volume caused by subclinical RV dysfunction.

Right heart catheterization in CTED often reveals either normal resting hemodynamics or borderline PH (mPA of 20–24 mm Hg with pulmonary vascular resistance of 2–3 Wood units). With exercise, there is an increased mPA/cardiac output slope, an exaggerated increase in mPA to greater than 30 to 35 mm Hg, and no or an inadequate decrease in pulmonary vascular resistance.[28] Patients with CTED generally have more preserved exercise capacity than patients with CTEPH and do not develop overt right

heart failure with exercise.[29] Apart from continued anticoagulation, limited medical therapy options exist for CTED, but pulmonary endarterectomy and balloon pulmonary angioplasty improve symptoms and exercise capacity in patients with CTED. Life-long chronic anticoagulation is recommended in all patients with CTED.[30]

An invasive cardiopulmonary exercise test (iCPET) combines gas exchange analysis obtained on the CPET examination with an exercise right heart catheterization.[27] iCPET, therefore, adds the ability to assess for exercise-induced PH in these patients. Patients with exercise-induced PH are grouped with those who have CTEPH at rest.

Persistent postpulmonary embolism dyspnea or "all others with postpulmonary embolism syndrome"
Although CTED and CTEPH (including exercise-induced PAH) have well-defined diagnostic criteria, only a minority of patients with persistent dyspnea and functional limitation after an acute PE meet these criteria.[31] A significant proportion of patients with PE with persistent symptoms are not found to have CTED or CTEPH and are classified as "all others with post-PE syndrome."[12,18] The authors believe these patients more accurately constitute "post-PE syndrome" and can be said to have "persistent post-PE dyspnea." It is defined as residual dyspnea, functional limitations, and poor quality of life at least 3 months

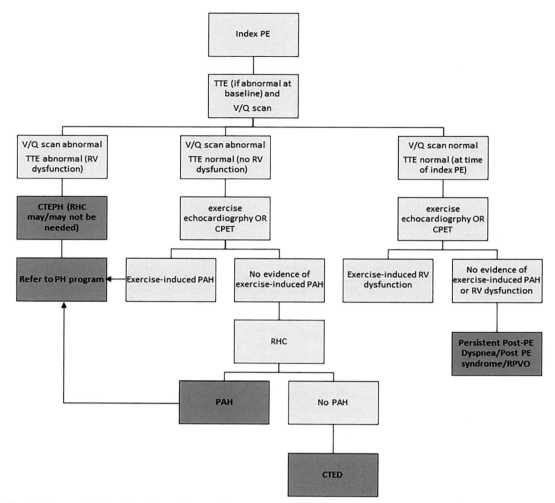

Fig. 2. Diagnostic algorithm for evaluation of persistent dyspnea and functional limitations after acute PE. RHC, right heart catheterization; RPVO, residual pulmonary vascular obstruction; TTE, transthoracic echocardiography.

after an acute PE episode. In the absence of identified cause, symptoms and functional limitations in these patients can be attributed to deconditioning.[32] Exercise testing with treadmill study or CPET can be used to quantify these limitations. Although exercise therapy would be expected to help such patients, in the absence of evidence-based literature, a formal exercise program, such as cardiac rehabilitation, is not usually covered by most payers in this scenario.[33]

Anticoagulation Therapy
Choice of an anticoagulant
For most patients with PE, including those with cancer-associated PE, direct-acting oral anticoagulant (DOAC) medications are the mainstays of treatment.[1] DOACs are safe and effective for treating all VTE except patients with

antiphospholipid syndrome, heparin-induced thrombocytopenia, or venous thrombosis at unusual sites, such as splanchnic vein thrombosis. In such cases, vitamin K antagonists (VKA) are preferred.[1]

In cancer-associated PE, DOACs and Lovenox are considered superior to VKA. In those with non-cancer-associated PE, VKA and DOACs are deemed equivalent in efficacy. DOACs also have limited efficacy data in patients with CTED/CTEPH but are often used off-label in this population.

Duration of anticoagulation
The duration of anticoagulation in PE is often based on future risk of recurrence, and the presence of CTED/CTEPH in follow-up. As previously mentioned, CTED/CTEPH warrants lifelong anticoagulation.

VTE and, by extension, PE are considered "provoked" by a transient or persistent risk factor or "unprovoked" in the absence of any identifiable risk factors for VTE. In patients with low risk of recurrence—such as those with PE caused by surgery or nonsurgical transient risk factors like immobilization, pregnancy, or estrogen therapy—anticoagulation is initially recommended for 3 months. Anticoagulation may be discontinued at 3 months if no evidence of CTED/CTEPH is noted in follow-up.

In patients with cancer-associated VTE, anticoagulation is recommended for a minimum of 6 months or as long as active cancer is present.

Most patients with unprovoked PE generally have a high risk of recurrence and should therefore receive indefinite anticoagulation if their bleeding risk is not high. Tools such as HERDOO2 and HAS-BLED scores can help assess the competing risk of recurrent VTE with the risk of bleeding, respectively. The HERDOO2 rule is intended to guide treatment duration decisions for women with a first unprovoked VTE by assessing the following risk factors for recurrence: postthrombotic signs (hyperpigmentation, edema, or redness in either leg), d-dimer during therapy $\geq$250 µg/L, body mass index $\geq$30 kg/m^2, and age $\geq$65 years. If none or one of these risk factors is present, anticoagulation may be discontinued after short-term treatment, even in those with unprovoked PE.[34] The HAS-BLED score estimates the risk of major bleeding among atrial fibrillation patients by incorporating uncontrolled hypertension, renal disease, liver disease, stroke history, prior major bleeding or predisposition to bleeding, labile international normalized ratio, age $\geq$65 years, medications that predispose bleeding, and alcohol use. Patients with 3 or more risk factors have a high risk of major bleeding (5.8%–9.1% in the study cohort).[35] The authors suggest using these tools

as an adjunct to clinical judgment and shared decision making. Tritschler and colleagues[1] recently proposed an algorithm to navigate anticoagulation decisions that balance the risk of recurrence and the risk of bleeding. Table 1 summarizes the proposed duration of anticoagulation in various clinical scenarios.

Thrombophilia testing

Appropriate testing for inherited thrombophilia can be done at follow-up. However, most patients with VTE should not be tested for thrombophilia owing to the lack of clinical usefulness and limited benefit. Most patients with inherited thrombophilia can be identified based on the patient's personal and family history of VTE, and testing is usually not required.

Factors associated with an inherited thrombophilia include VTE at a young age (<40–50 years), a strong family history of VTE, VTE in conjunction with weak provoking factors at a young age, recurrent VTE, and VTE in an unusual site (eg, cerebral or splanchnic veins).

Thrombophilia testing should not be performed at the time of a VTE event or while a patient is receiving anticoagulation. It should be performed 2 weeks after discontinuing warfarin, or 2 days for DOACs and heparin. However, it should only be undertaken if a management strategy would be impacted by it. The duration of anticoagulation is based mainly on the "provoked" or "unprovoked" status of VTE/PE, as mentioned previously. Patients with provoked VTE, even those with homozygous factor V Leiden, prothrombin gene mutations, or deficiencies of protein S, C, or antithrombin, do not require lifelong anticoagulation.

The goal of thrombophilia testing should be to aid decision making regarding future VTE prophylaxis, guide testing of family members,

Table 1 Author's proposed duration of anticoagulation			
PE Category			Duration of anticoagulation
Cancer associated PE			At least 6 mo OR until cancer is active
Subsegmental PE with low risk of recurrence			Clinical surveillance or 3 mo
PE Provoked by transient risk factor			3 mo
Unprovoked PE	Men	Low-moderate bleeding risk	Indefinite
		High-bleeding risk	3–6 mo
	Women	High recurrence risk with low-moderate bleeding risk	Indefinite
		Low recurrence risk	3–6 mo

Abbreviation: PE, pulmonary embolism.

and determine the cause of severe or fatal VTE. Test results alone should not be used to decide on the duration of anticoagulation therapy, as most VTE recurrence risk tools do not incorporate thrombophilia test results into their risk stratification schemes.[36] Table 2 summarizes common indications for thrombophilia workup.

Inferior vena cava filter
Although IVC filters decrease PE risk in patients with a contraindication to anticoagulation, they are also associated with an IVC perforation, filter migration, fracture, and thrombosis.[37] The Food and Drug Administration recommends removing IVC filters as soon as protection is no longer needed,[38] but retrieval rates remain low, with only a third of filters being removed.[39] A select group of patients may benefit from an IVC filter if potential long-term complications can be avoided: those with high-risk submassive PE with large, proximal DVTs who are at risk of cardiopulmonary compromise and have prohibitive bleeding risk from anticoagulation.[40] There should be a continued assessment of risk versus benefit of IVC filter at each follow-up visit, where the post-PE clinic has an important role. When no longer indicated, patients should be promptly referred for filter removal. When removal is attempted, filter removal has success rates ranging from 84% to 94%, and filters that could not be removed had higher dwell times than those successfully retrieved (375 vs 96 days).[40] Therefore, when indicated, early removal should be practiced.

Table 2
Indications to consider thrombophilia workup

Testing for inherited thrombophilia should be considered in the following situations, if results would change management in times of increased risk

After first VTE, in these scenarios:
- VTE provoked by weak trigger (minor surgery, prolonged air travel), in young patient with strong family history
- Unprovoked VTE
- VTE in unusual site (cerebral/CNS veins, splanchnic veins)
- Female patient of reproductive age and planning for future pregnancy or contraception may be impacted

After recurrent VTE, especially at young age

If family members have strong history of VTE, consider testing female relatives of childbearing age

Adapted from Connors 2017.

SUMMARY

The long-term management of PE requires focused and coordinated care that encompasses anticoagulation management, evaluation and management of complications, such as post-PE syndrome, and addressing thrombophilia testing and IVC filters. A dedicated long-term outpatient follow-up clinic streamlines the various aspects of care to potentially avoid complications and improve patients' quality of life.

CLINICS CARE POINTS

- When patients are seen for acute pulmonary embolism inpatient it would be best to ensure timely outpatient follow-up for long-term management.
- Anticoagulants management, complications of PE, thrombophilia testing and IVC filters need to be addressed in follow-up visits.

DISCLOSURE

All authors have no relevant disclosures related to this article.

REFERENCES

1. Tritschler T, Kraaijpoel N, Le Gal G, et al. Venous Thromboembolism: Advances in Diagnosis and Treatment. JAMA 2018;320(15):1583–94.
2. Turetz M, Sideris AT, Friedman OA, et al. Epidemiology, Pathophysiology, and Natural History of Pulmonary Embolism. Semin Intervent Radiol 2018; 35(2):92–8.
3. Tagalakis V, Patenaude V, Kahn SR, et al. Incidence of and mortality from venous thromboembolism in a real-world population: the Q-VTE Study Cohort. Am J Med 2013;126(9):832.e13-21.
4. Lang IM. Chronic Thromboembolic Pulmonary Hypertension — Not So Rare after All. N Engl J Med 2004;350(22):2236–8.
5. Tavoly M, Wik HS, Sirnes PA, et al. The impact of post-pulmonary embolism syndrome and its possible determinants. Thromb Res 2018;171:84–91.
6. den Exter PL, van der Hulle T, Lankeit M, et al. Long-term clinical course of acute pulmonary embolism. Blood Rev 2013;27(4):185–92.
7. Klok FA, Mos IC, Broek L, et al. Risk of arterial cardiovascular events in patients after pulmonary embolism. Blood 2009;114(8):1484–8.
8. Klok FA, Zondag W, van Kralingen KW, et al. Patient Outcomes after Acute Pulmonary Embolism. Am J Respir Crit Care Med 2010;181(5):501–6.

9. Lori-Ann Linkins PTC, Douketis JD. Clinical Impact of Bleeding in Patients Taking Oral Anticoagulant Therapy for Venous Thromboembolism. Ann Intern Med 2003;139(11):893–900.

10. Pengo V, Lensing AWA, Prins MH, et al. Incidence of Chronic Thromboembolic Pulmonary Hypertension after Pulmonary. Embolism 2004;350(22):2257–64.

11. Prandoni P, Noventa F, Ghirarduzzi A, et al. The risk of recurrent venous thromboembolism after discontinuing anticoagulation in patients with acute proximal deep vein thrombosis or pulmonary embolism. A prospective cohort study in 1,626 patients. Haematologica 2007;92(2):199–205.

12. Sista AK, Klok FA. Late outcomes of pulmonary embolism: The post-PE syndrome. Thromb Res 2018;164: 157–62.

13. Tapson VF, Platt DM, Xia F, et al. Monitoring for Pulmonary Hypertension Following Pulmonary Embolism: The INFORM Study. Am J Med 2016;129(9): 978–985 e2.

14. Rivera-Lebron B, McDaniel M, Ahrar K, et al. Diagnosis, Treatment and Follow Up of Acute Pulmonary Embolism: Consensus Practice from the PERT Consortium. Clin Appl Thromb Hemost 2019;25. 1076029619853037.

15. Klok FA, Cohn DM, Middeldorp S, et al. Quality of life after pulmonary embolism: validation of the PEmb-QoL Questionnaire. J Thromb Haemost 2010;8(3):523–32.

16. Boon GJAM, Barco S, Bertoletti L, et al. Measuring functional limitations after venous thromboembolism: Optimization of the Post-VTE Functional Status (PVFS) Scale. Thromb Res 2020;190:45–51.

17. McHorney CA, Ware JE Jr, Lu JF, et al. The MOS 36-item Short-Form Health Survey (SF-36): III. Tests of data quality, scaling assumptions, and reliability across diverse patient groups. Med Care 1994;32(1):40–66.

18. Klok FA, van der Hulle T, den Exter PL, et al. The post-PE syndrome: a new concept for chronic complications of pulmonary embolism. Blood Rev 2014;28(6):221–6.

19. Boon G, Bogaard HJ, Klok FA. Essential aspects of the follow-up after acute pulmonary embolism: An illustrated review. Research and practice in thrombosis and haemostasis 2020;4(6):958–68.

20. Galie N, Humbert M, Vachiery JL, et al. 2015 ESC/ERS Guidelines for the diagnosis and treatment of pulmonary hypertension: The Joint Task Force for the Diagnosis and Treatment of Pulmonary Hypertension of the European Society of Cardiology (ESC) and the European Respiratory Society (ERS): Endorsed by: Association for European Paediatric and Congenital Cardiology (AEPC), International Society for Heart and Lung Transplantation (ISHLT). Eur Heart J 2016;37(1):67–119.

21. Kim NH, Delcroix M, Jenkins DP, et al. Chronic thromboembolic pulmonary hypertension. J Am Coll Cardiol 2013;62(25 Suppl):D92–9.

22. Ruan W, Yap JJ, Quah KK, et al. Clinical Updates on the Diagnosis and Management of Chronic Thromboembolic Pulmonary Hypertension. Ann Acad Med Singap 2020;49(5):320–30.

23. Lisbona R, Kreisman H, Novales-Diaz J, et al. Perfusion lung scanning: differentiation of primary from thromboembolic pulmonary hypertension. AJR Am J Roentgenol 1985;144(1):27–30.

24. Powe JE, Palevsky HI, McCarthy KE, et al. Pulmonary arterial hypertension: value of perfusion scintigraphy. Radiology 1987;164(3):727–30.

25. Mahmud E, Madani MM, Kim NH, et al. Chronic Thromboembolic Pulmonary Hypertension: Evolving Therapeutic Approaches for Operable and Inoperable Disease. J Am Coll Cardiol 2018;71(21):2468–86.

26. Guazzi M, Bandera F, Ozemek C, et al. Cardiopulmonary Exercise Testing: What Is its Value? J Am Coll Cardiol 2017;70(13):1618–36.

27. Maron BA, Cockrill BA, Waxman AB, et al. The invasive cardiopulmonary exercise test. Circulation 2013;127(10):1157–64.

28. Guth S, Wiedenroth CB, Rieth A, et al. Exercise right heart catheterisation before and after pulmonary endarterectomy in patients with chronic thromboembolic disease. Eur Respir J 2018;52(3). https://doi.org/10.1183/13993003.00458-2018.

29. Taboada D, Pepke-Zaba J, Jenkins DP, et al. Outcome of pulmonary endarterectomy in symptomatic chronic thromboembolic disease. Eur Respir J 2014;44(6):1635–45.

30. Pugliese SC, Kawut SM. The Post-Pulmonary Embolism Syndrome: Real or Ruse? Annals of the American Thoracic Society 2019;16(7):811–4.

31. Sista AK, Miller LE, Kahn SR, et al. Persistent right ventricular dysfunction, functional capacity limitation, exercise intolerance, and quality of life impairment following pulmonary embolism: Systematic review with meta-analysis. Vasc Med 2017;22(1):37–43.

32. Kahn SR, Hirsch AM, Akaberi A, et al. Functional and Exercise Limitations After a First Episode of Pulmonary Embolism: Results of the ELOPE Prospective Cohort Study. Chest 2017;151(5):1058–68. https://doi.org/10.1016/j.chest.2016.11.030. Epub 20161206. PubMed PMID: 27932051.

33. Jervan Ø, Haukeland-Parker S, Gleditsch J, et al. The effects of exercise training in patients with persistent dyspnoea after pulmonary embolism: a randomized controlled trial. Chest. 2023. Epub 20230504. https://doi.org/10.1016/j.chest.2023.04.042. PubMed PMID: 37149257.

34. Rodger MA, Le Gal G, Anderson DR, et al. Validating the HERDOO2 rule to guide treatment duration for women with unprovoked venous thrombosis: multinational prospective cohort management study. BMJ 2017;356:j1065.

35. Lip GY, Frison L, Halperin JL, et al. Comparative validation of a novel risk score for predicting

bleeding risk in anticoagulated patients with atrial fibrillation: the HAS-BLED (Hypertension, Abnormal Renal/Liver Function, Stroke, Bleeding History or Predisposition, Labile INR, Elderly, Drugs/Alcohol Concomitantly) score. J Am Coll Cardiol 2011;57(2):173–80.

36. Connors JM. Thrombophilia Testing and Venous Thrombosis. N Engl J Med 2017;377(12): 1177–87.

37. Morrow KL, Bena J, Lyden SP, et al. Factors predicting failure of retrieval of inferior vena cava filters. Journal of vascular surgery Venous and lymphatic disorders 2020;8(1):44–52.

38. Shah M, Alnabelsi T, Patil S, et al. IVC filters-Trends in placement and indications, a study of 2 populations. Medicine 2017;96(12):e6449.

39. Salei A, Raborn J, Manapragada PP, et al. Effect of a dedicated inferior vena cava filter retrieval program on retrieval rates and number of patients lost to follow-up. Diagn Interventional Radiol 2020;26(1):40–4.

40. Marron RM, Rali P, Hountras P, et al. Inferior Vena Cava Filters: Past, Present, and Future. Chest 2020. https://doi.org/10.1016/j.chest.2020.08.002.

APPENDIX 1: THE PULMONARY EMBOLISM QUALITY OF LIFE QUESTIONNAIRE

Questionnaire:

After having a pulmonary embolism

Instructions on how to answer:

Answer every question by marking the answer as indicated. If you are unsure about how to answer a question, please give the best answer you can.

These questions are about your *lungs*. The information you give should describe how you feel. You can also indicate how capable you are of carrying out your normal activities.

1. During the *past 4 weeks*, how often have you had any of the following symptoms from your lungs? *(circle 1 answer on each line)*

	Every day	Several times a week	About once a week	Less than once a week	Never
Pain behind or between the shoulder blades?	1	2	3	4	5
Pain on or in the chest?	1	2	3	4	5
Pain in the back?	1	2	3	4	5
Sensation of pressure?	1	2	3	4	5
Feeling that there is "still something there"?	1	2	3	4	5
"Burning sensation" in the lungs?	1	2	3	4	5
"Nagging feeling" in the lungs?	1	2	3	4	5
Difficulty in breathing or breathlessness?	1	2	3	4	5

2. At what time of day are your lung symptoms most intense? (circle one answer)
   1. On waking
   2. At midday
   3. At the end of the day
   4. During the night
   5. At any time of the day
   6. Never

3. Compared to 1 year ago, how would you rate the condition of your lungs in general now? (circle one answer)
   1. Much better now than 1 year ago
   2. Somewhat better now than 1 year ago
   3. About the same now as 1 year ago
   4. Somewhat worse now than 1 year ago
   5. Much worse now than 1 year ago
   6. I did not have any problems with my lungs

4. The following items are about activities that you might do in a typical day. *Do your lung symptoms now limit you* in these activities? If so, how much? *(circle one answer on each line)*

	I do not work	YES, limited a lot	YES, limited a little	NO, not limited at all
a. Daily activities at work	0	1	2	3
b. Daily activities at home (eg, housework, ironing, doing odd jobs/repairs around the house, gardening, etc....)		1	2	3
c. Social or activities (such as traveling, going to the cinema, parties, shopping)		1	2	3
d. Vigorous activities, such as running, lifting heavy objects, participating in strenuous sports		1	2	3
e. Moderate activities, such as moving a table, vacuuming, swimming, or cycling		1	2	3
f. Lifting or carrying groceries		1	2	3

(continued on next page)

(continued)

g. Climbing several flights of stairs	1	2	3
h. Climbing one flight of stairs	1	2	3
i. Bending, kneeling, or squatting	1	2	3
j. Walking more than half a mile	1	2	3
k. Walking a couple of hundred yards	1	2	3
l. Walking about one hundred yards	1	2	3
m. Washing or dressing yourself	1	2	3

5. During *the past 4 weeks*, have you had any of the following problems with your work or other regular daily activities *as a result of your lung symptoms*? *(circle one answer on each line)*

	YES	NO
a. Cut down the amount of time you spent on work or other activities	1	2
b. Accomplished less than you would like	1	2
c. Were limited in the kind of work or other activities	1	2
d. Had difficulty performing the work or other activities (eg, it took extra effort)	1	2

6. During the *past 4 weeks*, to what extent have your *lung symptoms* interfered with your normal social activities with family, friends, neighbors, or groups? *(circle one answer)*

1. Not at all   4. Quite a bit
2. Slightly   5. Extremely
3. Moderately

7. How much pain around your shoulder blades/pain in your chest have you experienced during the past 4 weeks? *(circle one answer)*

1. None   4. Quite a bit
2. Very slight   5. Serious
3. Slight   6. Very serious

8. How much breathlessness have you experienced in the past 4 weeks? *(circle one answer)*

1. None   4. Quite a bit
2. Very slight   5. Serious
3. Slight   6. Very serious

9. These questions are about how you feel and how things have been with you *during the past 4 weeks as a result of your lung symptoms*. For each question, please give the one answer that comes closest to the way you have been feeling. How much of the time during the *past 4 weeks (circle one answer on each line)*

	All of the time	Most of the time	A good bit of the time	Some of the time	A little of the time	None of the time

(continued on next page)

(continued)						
Were you worried about having another pulmonary embolism?	1	2	3	4	5	6
Did you feel irritable?	1	2	3	4	5	6
Would you have been worried if you had to stop taking anticoagulant medication?	1	2	3	4	5	6
Did you become emotional more readily?	1	2	3	4	5	6
Did it bother you that you became emotional more quickly?	1	2	3	4	5	6
Were you depressed or in low spirits?	1	2	3	4	5	6
Did you feel that you were a burden to your family and friends?	1	2	3	4	5	6
Were you afraid to exert yourself?	1	2	3	4	5	6
Did you feel limited in taking a trip?	1	2	3	4	5	6
Were you afraid of being alone?	1	2	3	4	5	6

Legend to the Appendix: Higher scores indicate worse outcome. Scores for all dimensions are calculated by the sum of the scores for each item of the dimension divided by the number of the items. Questions 1, 4, 5, and 9 are reversed scored. Questions 2 and 3 provide descriptive information.

Thank you very much for your cooperation.

Please return the questionnaire in the enclosed prepaid envelope or give it to your doctor.

(Adapted from FA Klok et al 2010.)

APPENDIX 2: THE POST–VENOUS THROMBOEMBOLISM FUNCTIONAL STATUS—PATIENT SELF-REPORT

How much are you currently affected in your everyday life by the VTE? Please indicate which one of the following statements applies to you most. *Please tick only one box at a time.*	*Corresponding PVFS scale grade if the box is ticked*
I have no limitations in my everyday life and no symptoms, pain, or anxiety related to the VTE.	0
I have negligible limitations in my everyday life, as I can perform all usual duties/activities, although I still have persistent symptoms, pain, or anxiety.	1
I suffer from limitations in my everyday life, as I occasionally need to avoid or reduce usual duties/activities or need to spread these over time due to symptoms, pain, or anxiety. I am, however, able to perform all activities without any assistance.	2
I suffer from limitations in my everyday life, as I am not able to perform all usual duties/activities due to symptoms, pain, or anxiety. I am, however, able to take care of myself without any assistance.	3
I suffer from severe limitations in my everyday life: I am not able to take care of myself, and therefore, I am dependent on nursing care and/or assistance from another person due to symptoms, pain, or anxiety.	4

(Adapted from Boon et al 2020.)

Patient self-report flow chart for the Post-VTE functional Scale

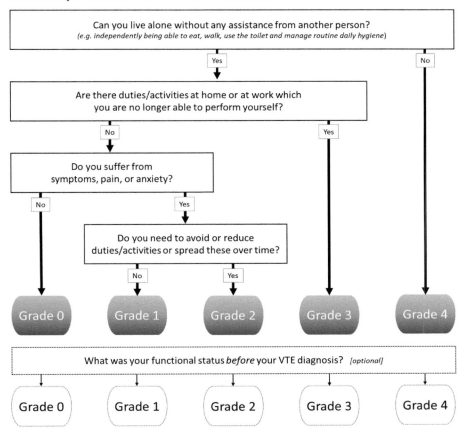

The Intersection of Pulmonary Vascular Disease and Hypoxia-Inducible Factors

Madathilparambil V. Suresh, PhD[a],
Vikas Aggarwal, MD, MPH[b,c],
Krishnan Raghavendran, MD[a,*]

KEYWORDS

• HIF 1 alpha • Pulmonary hypertension • Pulmonary vascular disease

---

KEY POINTS

- Hypoxia-inducible factors (HIFs) are a family of nuclear transcription factors that serve as the master regulator of the adaptive response to hypoxia.
- In pulmonary hypertension, there appears to be a clear role for mitochondrial abnormalities related to reactive oxygen species and subsequent activation of both HIF-1α and HIF2α.
- Despite a clear mechanistic role for both HIF 1α and 2α in pulmonary vascular diseases including PH, a succesful translation into a defintive therapeutic modality has not been accomplished to date.

HYPOXIA-INDUCIBLE FACTORS

Hypoxia-inducible factors (HIFs) are a family of nuclear transcription factors that serve as the master regulator of the adaptive response to hypoxia. These transcription factors, including HIF-1, 2, and 3, control the transcription of numerous genes involved in metabolism, angiogenesis, erythropoiesis, and other adaptations to hypoxia. Hypoxia-inducible factor 1 (HIF-1) is composed of HIF-1 alpha and HIF-1 beta subunits (Fig. 1). The basis of oxygen sensing for all 3 HIFs is the hydroxylation of proline residues in the oxygen-dependent degradation domain by dioxygenase prolyl-hydroxylase (PHD).[1–3] PHDs require an iron cofactor for their catalysis and, therefore, also function as sensors for intracellular iron.[4] Additionally, hydroxylation of the proline residues serves as an interaction scaffold for the recognition of the von Hippel-Lindau-containing E3-ligase complex and the following degradation by the proteasome but hydroxylation of the asparagine residue leads to inhibition of CREB-cAMP response element-binding protein (CBP)/p300 recruitment.[5,6]

In the setting of hypoxia, HIFs are stabilized and translocate to the nucleus where they heterodimerize with the aryl hydrocarbon nuclear translocator, also known as HIF-1β.[7] This heterodimer complex binds to the core DNA sequence 5'-TACGTG-3' within the hypoxia response element (HRE) of target promoters in conjunction with the p300/CBP complex and other coactivators.[8,9] HIF-1α is the most prominent isoform implicated in the pathogenesis of inflammatory lung injury.[10] It binds to the core DNA sequence within the HRE of target promoters and causes the activation of more than 200 genes involved in various pathways, including inflammation and angiogenesis.[11]

---

[a] Division of Acute Care Surgery, Department of Surgery, University of Michigan, Ann Arbor, MI, USA; [b] Division of Cardiology (Frankel Cardiovascular Center), Department of Internal Medicine, University of Michigan, Ann Arbor, MI, USA; [c] Section of Cardiology, Department of Internal Medicine, Veterans Affairs Medical Center, Ann Arbor, MI, USA
* Corresponding author. 1C340 University Hospital, SPC 5033, 1500 East Medical Center Drive, Ann Arbor, MI 48109-5033.
E-mail address: kraghave@umich.edu

Intervent Cardiol Clin 12 (2023) 443–452
https://doi.org/10.1016/j.iccl.2023.03.010
2211-7458/23/© 2023 Elsevier Inc. All rights reserved.

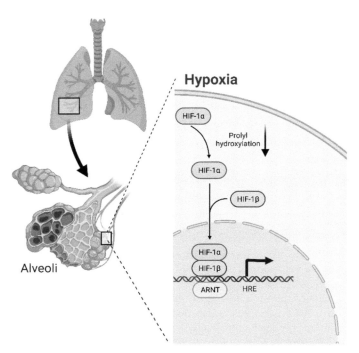

Hypoxia

Alveoli

Fig. 1. HIF signaling pathway in hypoxic conditions: Under normoxic conditions, HIF-1/2α is stabilized by PHDs in the presence of O_2. Under the normoxic stage, ubiquitination is enhanced by the von Hippel-Lindau tumor suppressor protein (VHL) and targets HIF-1/2α for degradation. However, during hypoxic conditions, PHDs and FIH are unable to hydroxylate HIF-α subunits, which are translocated into the nucleus, resulting in dimerization of HIF-1α and HIF1β, recruitment of p300 and CBP, and ultimately, binding to HREs at target genes to cause activation. This complex thereby activates specific genes, which will further trigger pathological activities.

It is important to remember that nonhypoxic factors such as growth factors, inflammatory mediators, and metabolic byproducts (eg, succinate) also regulate HIF molecules. The nature of these interactions is complex and often bidirectional.

In the lung, HIF orchestrates multiple inflammatory pathways and signaling. They have been reported to have a major role in the initiation and progression of acute lung injury (ALI), chronic obstructive pulmonary disease, pulmonary fibrosis (PF), and pulmonary hypertension.

Interaction of Hypoxia-Inducible Factor and Inflammation, Growth Factors, and Vaso-Reactive Molecules

There is a well-known link between hypoxia and inflammation. Prominent among factors other than hypoxia that activate HIF-1α is nuclear factor Kappa B (NF-κB). This transcription factor is controlled through the IkB (inhibitor of NF-κB) kinases, inhibitor of nuclear factor kB kinase alpha (IKKα) and inhibitor of nuclear factor kB kinase beta (IKKβ). Once these kinases are phosphorylated, which occurs under hypoxic conditions, they phosphorylate IkBα-β, causing its degradation and the release of NF-κB.[12,13] NF-κB, in turn, can upregulate the transcription of HIFs.[13–15] HIF-1α participates in a negative feedback loop by inducing the transforming growth factor-β (TGF-β)-activated kinase 1 (TAK1) (TAK)–TAB complex and cell division protein kinase 6 (CDK6) to sequester

NF-κB.[16] In addition to the IKK/NF-κB pathway, HIFs also modulate the P13 Kinase-phosphoinositide-3-kinase/akt-protein kinase B (PI3K/AKT) pathway, of which NF-κB is a downstream effector.[17] HIF-1α, as a result, is directly involved in the regulation of a wide range of proinflammatory proteins, including interleukin-1β (IL-1β), IL-6, macrophage inflammatory proteins (MIP-1), tumor necrosis factor (TNF-α), hydrogen peroxide, and prostaglandins in alveolar macrophages (AM).[18–22] A bidirectional relationship, therefore, exists between HIF-1α and NF-κB.

Our laboratory and others have characterized the role of the alveolar epithelium in hypoxic inflammation. Type II alveolar epithelial cells (AECs) are a significant source of chemotactic factors, such as CCL20 (chemokine ligand 20), CCL2, and C-X-C motif chemokine ligand 1 (CXCL1), which serve as recruitment signals for circulating leukocytes and adhesive factors for leukocyte extravasation, such as intercellular adhesion molecule 1, and vascular cell adhesion protein 1.[23–26] Similar to AM, Type II AECs produce many proinflammatory mediators, including MIP-2, granulocyte-macrophage colony-stimulating factor, IL-6, and IL-1β.[24,27,28] Interestingly, recent study has revealed an anti-inflammatory mechanism involving HIFs in regulating extracellular adenosine, a metabolite involved in dampening the inflammatory response. HIF-1α regulation of heme oxygenase-1 (HO-1) has also been identified as an important anti-inflammatory pathway.[29]

Nitric oxide (NO) is known to play a major role in the maintenance of vascular tone including the pulmonary circulation. Studies indicate that NO effects on pulmonary arterial endothelial cells are mediated through HIF. For example, lower levels of NO caused by the deletion of endothelial NO synthase cause stabilization of HIF-1α. Additionally, endothelin-1 (ET-1), a potent vasoconstrictor also stabilizes HIF-1α, likely mediated through increased calcium signaling and the extracellular signal regulated kinases (ERK) pathway.[30] This is particularly evident in the pulmonary artery smooth muscles and involves intermediate generation of reactive oxygen species (ROS). Finally, HIF also regulates the level of ET-1[31] suggesting a bidirectional loop similar to the one seen with acute inflammation.

There are several growth factors reported to be directly or indirectly involved in the regulation of HIFs. Prominent among them are estradiol and bone morphogenetic protein (BMP). Estradiol negative regulation of ET-1 is mediated through HIF-1α and additionally reduces levels of HIF-2α by promoting its degradation.[32] Both these activities center around smooth muscles and vascular endothelium. BMP has a myriad number of functions in the regulation of HIF. Most notable among them is the negative regulation of HIF-2α in the pulmonary artery endothelial cells (PAECs) mediated through proteins suppressor of mothers against decapentaplegic 1 and 5.[33]

EFFECT OF HYPOXIA-INDUCIBLE FACTOR ON CELLULAR METABOLISM

HIFs curtail functions associated with oxygen usage, shunting metabolism toward the glycolytic pathway. It was previously thought that the glycolytic pathway was used under hypoxic conditions because oxygen is limiting. However, studies show that during hypoxia (1% O_2), HIF-1α (−/−) cells do not finish oxidative phosphorylation. These cells eventually undergo apoptosis due to excessive ROS.[34,35] Notably, HIFs reduce ROS production formed as a byproduct of the electron transport chain. The aerobic glycolysis reaction favored by HIF signaling is called the Warburg effect.

Glycolysis is modulated under hypoxic conditions through HIF-controlled upregulation of the glycolytic enzymes aldolase A, phosphoglycerate kinase 1, enolase 1, phosphofructokinase 2, and pyruvate kinase, all of which have been found to contain HREs within their promoter regions.[36–38] HIF-1α also upregulates pyruvate dehydrogenase kinase and lactate dehydrogenase.[39] Glucose transporter 1 (GLUT1), a vital glucose transporter, is upregulated by HIF-1α under hypoxic conditions to promote glycolysis further.[40] Inflammation has also been shown to trigger the switch to aerobic glycolysis through an AKT-mTOR-HIF-1α pathway mediated by the α-glucan receptor dectin-1 in response to immunogenic challenge.[41] In addition, Eckle and colleagues demonstrated, with models of ventilator-induced ALI, that HIF-1α is stabilized even in normoxia, promoting glycolysis, the tricarboxylic acid cycle, and preventing worsening of lung injury.[42]

PHD activity is blocked by succinate and fumarate, stabilizing HIF-1α activity.[43] Succinate, specifically in macrophages, stabilizes HIF-1α and is a predominant regulator of acute inflammation, mediated by IL-1β.[18] Plasma level of succinate is reported to predict mortality in critically injured trauma patients.[44] Finally, HIFs downregulate the biosynthesis of mitochondria while simultaneously increasing mitophagy.[45,46] The enzymatic regulation of the metabolic pathways by HIF in the context of pulmonary hypertension is discussed in detail below.

In the context of pulmonary hypertension, there seems to be a clear role for mitochondrial abnormalities related to ROS and subsequent activation of HIF-1α specifically in pulmonary vasculature.[47]

ROLE OF HYPOXIA-INDUCIBLE FACTOR IN VASCULAR GROWTH, SMOOTH MUSCLE PROLIFERATION, AND VASCULAR REMODELING

HIFs upregulate genes involved in oxygen delivery. This effect manifests in the rapid angiogenesis and vascularization promoted in hypoxic tissues. The arterial vasculature is composed of 3 layers. The tunica intima is the innermost layer and is composed of endothelial cells. Hypoxia stimulates hypertrophy and subendothelial edema in the tunica intima.[48,49] Hypoxic stress has also been associated with increased endothelial cell barrier permeability, possibly due to alterations of actin fibers and increased secretions of various vasoconstrictive and promitogenic factors. Vascular endothelium growth factor (VEGF), a prototypical promitogenic factor, is a potent angiogenic agent excreted in response to hypoxia by endothelial and nonendothelial cells including AEC and AM.[50–52] HIF-1α in endothelial cells regulates the production of stromal-derived factor, which recruits stem cells to areas of hypoxia and vascularization.[53] Recent evidence also suggests a role for HIFs in releasing the factors thrombospondin-1 and ET-1, which are involved in vasoconstriction and vascular remodeling.[54,55] Furthermore, HIFs promote vascular remodeling and alveolarization in various models of lung injury and prolonged hypoxia.[56–60] These changes are also stimulated by inflammatory cytokines such as IL-6 and the recruitment of cells of monocytic lineage, both of which have been shown to act synergistically with hypoxia.[61–63]

A notable effect on the pulmonary arterial smooth muscle is the interactive regulation between adhesion molecule CD146 and HIF-1α through an NF-kB pathway. CD146, a junction molecule in the vascular endothelium, is stably expressed across the vasculature in most major organs, including the pulmonary vasculature. It has demonstrable pleiotropic effects that include the regulation of vascular permeability, angiogenesis, and leukocyte transmigration.[64] Recently, it has been shown that the expression of CD146 in smooth muscle correlates with the severity of pulmonary hypertension.[65] Moreover, this expression was directly mediated by HIF-1α. Finally, the authors were able to show that the disruption of the HIF-1α-CD146 axis markedly attenuated pulmonary hypertension.[65]

ROLE OF HYPOXIA-INDUCIBLE FACTOR IN RIGHT VENTRICULAR REMODELING

Pulmonary arterial hypertension (PAH)-mediated secondary effects on the right ventricle and subsequent right heart failure are the primary determinants of mortality in patients with pulmonary hypertension. Right ventricular modeling because of pulmonary hypertension (PH) involves hyperplasia, hypertrophy of the cardiac myocytes, as well as extracellular matrix deposition. The regulation of right ventricular remodeling is, in part, controlled by HIF. The increased HIF-1α expression in the right ventricle in physiologically normal state[66] is exaggerated in multiple small animal models of pulmonary hypertension, including secondary effects of pulmonary embolism.[67] Interestingly, an increased expression of HIF-2 is associated with right ventricular dilatation without concomitant hypertrophy.[68] A summary of the literature suggests that while mild increases in both HIF-1α and HIF-2α expressions are associated with stable right ventricular function, a severe increase in HIF-1α and HIF-2α activation is associated with severe right heart dysfunction. Prolyl hydroxylase deletion (resulting in increased HIF-1α and HIF-2α levels) in mice causes significant right heart dilation and cardiomyopathy.[69]

ROLE OF HYPOXIA-INDUCIBLE FACTOR 1α IN PULMONARY HYPERTENSION

The complete role of HIF-1α in PH remains unclear and continues to be studied. Exhaustive review of this subject is presented elsewhere.[70] See Fig. 2 for details.[70] A summary of studies in animals and humans is provided below:

- The cellular sources of increased HIF-1α expression in lung tissue of PH patients are PAECs,[71,72] and pulmonary artery smooth muscle cells.[73,74]
- HIF signaling has been identified of mechanistic importance not only in PAH (group I PH) but also including PH associated with chronic high altitude exposure,[75] chronic obstructive pulmonary disease (COPD),[76] and PF[77] (group III PH). Increased expression of HIF-1α has been observed in lung tissues of patients with PAH,[78,79] chronic thromboembolic PH,[80] and idiopathic PF-associated PH.[71]
- In addition, neonatal patients with acute respiratory disease–associated PH also display increased circulating levels of HIF-1α.[81]
- HIF-1α and its target genes, VEGF and erythropoietin, are upregulated in peripheral blood cells of newborns with cyanosis and persistent PH, therefore representing early markers of generalized hypoxia.[82]
- Increases in circulating bone marrow–derived progenitor cells observed in PAH patients are regulated by HIF-1α–driven CXCL12 expression in PAECs.[83]
- The axis involving HIF-1α and junction molecule CD146 has been shown to drive the degree of pulmonary arterial hypertension in both murine studies as well as human correlates.[65]

ROLE OF HYPOXIA-INDUCIBLE FACTOR 2α IN PULMONARY HYPERTENSION

A summary of the mechanistic importance of HIF-2α in studies with rodents and human patients with pulmonary arterial hypertension is provided below:

- Increased expression of HIF-2α has been observed in children in PH associated with congenital diaphragmatic hernia and adults with PAH.[84]
- The major cellular source of HIF-2α is the pulmonary arterial endothelial cells.[85]

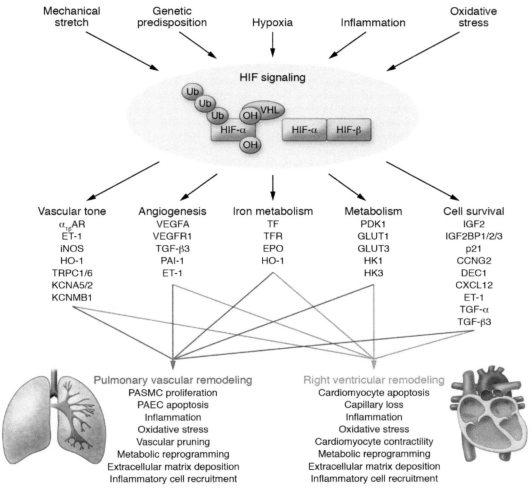

Fig. 2. Emerging concepts of HIF signaling in pulmonary hypertension. Emerging evidence shows that many pro-PH factors apart from hypoxia, such as inflammation, mechanical stretch, oxidative stress, and genetic predisposition, converge on HIF signaling pathways, causing alterations in vascular tone, angiogenesis, metabolism, and cell survival that subsequently lead to pulmonary vascular and right ventricular remodeling. CCNG2, cyclin-G2; DEC1, deleted in esophageal cancer 1; EPO, erythropoietin; HO-1, heme oxygenase-1; IGF2BP1, insulin-like growth factor 2 mRNA-binding protein 1; iNOS, inducible nitric oxide synthase; KCNA5, potassium voltage-gated channel, shaker-related subfamily, member 5; KCNMB1, calcium-activated potassium channel subunit beta-1; p21, cyclin-dependent kinase inhibitor 1; PAI-1, plasminogen activator inhibitor-1; PDK1, pyruvate dehydrogenase kinase 1; TF, transferrin; TFR, transferrin receptor; TRPC1, transient receptor potential canonical 1; VHL, von Hippel–Lindau tumor suppressor; $\alpha_{1\beta}$AR, $\alpha_1\beta$-adrenergic receptor. (See publication for other details.[70])

- HIF-2α, in addition to HIF-1α, also contributes to altered metabolic phenotype in the endothelial cells—the main effect includes increased "Warburg" effect (aerobic glycolysis).[86]
- HIF-2α expression is associated with an increased endothelial-mesenchymal transition.[85] This phenomenon is associated with increased neointima formation identified to be of importance in patients with idiopathic pulmonary arterial hypertension.

- Mice with heterogenous deletion of HIF-2α are protected from developing PH.[60]
- Mice with endothelial cell–specific deletion of HIF-2α develop PAH and right ventricular dilatation but not hypertrophy.[87]

THERAPEUTIC TARGETING OF HYPOXIA-INDUCIBLE FACTOR IN PULMONARY HYPERTENSION

a. *Animal studies:* Based on the presented experimental data outlined in the current article, it is clear that both HIF-1α and HIF-2α are mechanistically important in the pathogenesis of PH. Therapeutic strategies in animal models are summarized below:

- Digoxin, a drug used in heart failure, has been shown to suppress the accumulation of HIF-1α and subsequently prevented the induction of PH in chronically hypoxic mice.[88]
- Acriflavine, which inhibits both HIF-1α and HIF-2α, has similar therapeutic effects of preventing PH in chronically hypoxic mice.[89]
- Targeting of HIF-2 by small molecule inhibitor C76 has been shown to reverse the onset of PH in multiple animal models including SU5416 combined with hypoxia (SuHx) and monocrotaline (MCT) rats.[90]
- Suppression of HIF-2α signaling by antisense oligonucleotide protects the development of pulmonary arterial thickening following hypoxia.[91]
- A notable feature of transient HIF-2α inhibition was the hemodynamic response of the right heart was preserved without affecting the compensation to pressure overload.[92]

b. Human subject clinical trials involving HIF downstream pathway.

Although HIF has not been a target for human studies in PH thus far, oxidative stress has been targeted in a phase 2 study of Selonsertib (an inhibitor of apoptosis signal-regulating kinase 1) and has failed to show an overall improvement in PH.[93] A phase 3 study with bardoxolone methyl in scleroderma has also been completed, following some signals of efficacy in phase 2 clinical trial (NCT02036970). This drug induces the nuclear factor erythroid 2-related factor 2, a transcription factor that regulates antioxidant proteins, and suppresses the activation of the proinflammatory factor NF-κB. Although reports indicate that the study was completed in 2021, there are currently no publications available on the results of this clinical trial.

CLINICS CARE POINTS

- In the context of pulmonary hypertension, there appears to be a clear role for mitochondrial abnormalities related to reactive oxygen species and subsequent activation of both HIF-1α and HIF2α.
- Most of the HIF is generated either from pulmonary vasuclar endothelial cells or smotth muscles lining the vasculature.

- Though there appear to be a clear mechanistic role for both HIF 1α and 2α in pulmonary vascular diseases including PH, a succesful translation into a defintive therapeutic modality has not been accomplished to date.

DECLARATION OF INTERESTS

All authors have no relevant relationships to disclose.

REFERENCES

1. Jaakkola P, Mole DR, Tian YM, et al. Targeting of HIF-alpha to the von Hippel-Lindau ubiquitylation complex by O2-regulated prolyl hydroxylation. Science 2001;292(5516):468–72.
2. Masson N, Willam C, Maxwell PH, et al. Independent function of two destruction domains in hypoxia-inducible factor-alpha chains activated by prolyl hydroxylation. EMBO J 2001;20(18):5197–206.
3. Maynard MA, Qi H, Chung J, et al. Multiple splice variants of the human HIF-3 alpha locus are targets of the von Hippel-Lindau E3 ubiquitin ligase complex. J Biol Chem 2003;278(13):11032–40.
4. Xu MM, Wang J, Xie JX, et al. Regulation of iron metabolism by hypoxia-inducible factors. Sheng Li Xue Bao 2017;69(5):598–610.https://www.ncbi.nlm.nih.gov/pubmed/29063108.
5. Sang N, Fang J, Srinivas V, et al. Carboxyl-terminal transactivation activity of hypoxia-inducible factor 1 alpha is governed by a von Hippel-Lindau protein-independent, hydroxylation-regulated association with p300/CBP. Mol Cell Biol 2002;22(9):2984–92.
6. Lando D, Peet DJ, Whelan DA, et al. Asparagine hydroxylation of the HIF transactivation domain a hypoxic switch. Science 2002;295(5556):858–61.
7. Stolze I, Berchner-Pfannschmidt U, Freitag P, et al. Hypoxia-inducible erythropoietin gene expression in human neuroblastoma cells. Blood 2002;100(7):2623–8.
8. Arany Z, Huang LE, Eckner R, et al. An essential role for p300/CBP in the cellular response to hypoxia. Proc Natl Acad Sci U S A 1996;93(23):12969–73 (In eng) Available at: http://www.ncbi.nlm.nih.gov/pubmed/8917528.
9. Bhattacharya S, Michels CL, Leung MK, et al. Functional role of p35srj, a novel p300/CBP binding protein, during transactivation by HIF-1. Genes Dev 1999;13(1):64–75.
10. Shimoda LA, Semenza GL. HIF and the lung: role of hypoxia-inducible factors in pulmonary development and disease. Am J Respir Crit Care Med 2011;183(2):152–6.

11. Semenza GL. Oxygen sensing, hypoxia-inducible factors, and disease pathophysiology. Annu Rev Pathol 2014;9:47–71.
12. Hacker H, Karin M. Regulation and function of IKK and IKK-related kinases. Sci STKE 2006;2006(357):re13.
13. Rius J, Guma M, Schachtrup C, et al. NF-kappaB links innate immunity to the hypoxic response through transcriptional regulation of HIF-1alpha. Nature 2008;453(7196):807–11 (In eng).
14. Jiang H, Zhu YS, Xu H, et al. Inflammatory stimulation and hypoxia cooperatively activate HIF-1 {alpha} in bronchial epithelial cells: involvement of PI3K and NF-{kappa}B. Am J Physiol Lung Cell Mol Physiol 2010;298(5):L660–9 (In eng).
15. van Uden P, Kenneth NS, Rocha S. Regulation of hypoxia-inducible factor-1alpha by NF-kappaB. Biochem J 2008;412(3):477–84 (In eng).
16. Bandarra D, Biddlestone J, Mudie S, et al. HIF-1alpha restricts NF-kappaB-dependent gene expression to control innate immunity signals. Dis Model Mech 2015;8(2):169–81.
17. Zhang J, Guo H, Zhu JS, et al. Inhibition of phosphoinositide 3-kinase/Akt pathway decreases hypoxia inducible factor-1alpha expression and increases therapeutic efficacy of paclitaxel in human hypoxic gastric cancer cells. Oncol Lett 2014; 7(5):1401–8.
18. Tannahill GM, Curtis AM, Adamik J, et al. Succinate is an inflammatory signal that induces IL-1beta through HIF-1alpha. Nature 2013;496(7444):238–42.
19. VanOtteren GM, Standiford TJ, Kunkel SL, et al. Alterations of ambient oxygen tension modulate the expression of tumor necrosis factor and macrophage inflammatory protein-1 alpha from murine alveolar macrophages. Am J Respir Cell Mol Biol 1995;13(4):399–409 (In eng).
20. Wilhelm J, Sojkoví J, Herget J. Production of hydrogen peroxide by alveolar macrophages from rats exposed to subacute and chronic hypoxia. Physiol Res 1996;45(3):185–91 (In eng).
21. Compeau CG, Ma J, DeCampos KN, et al. In situ ischemia and hypoxia enhance alveolar macrophage tissue factor expression. Am J Respir Cell Mol Biol 1994;11(4):446–55 (In eng).
22. Fernandez-Bustamante A, Klawitter J, Wilson P, et al. Early increase in alveolar macrophage prostaglandin 15d-PGJ2 precedes neutrophil recruitment into lungs of cytokine-insufflated rats. Inflammation 2013;36(5):1030–40 (In eng).
23. Thorley AJ, Goldstraw P, Young A, et al. Primary human alveolar type II epithelial cell CCL20 (macrophage inflammatory protein-3alpha)-induced dendritic cell migration. Am J Respir Cell Mol Biol 2005;32(4):262–7 (In eng).
24. Suresh MV, Ramakrishnan SK, Thomas B, et al. Activation of hypoxia-inducible factor-1alpha in type 2 alveolar epithelial cell is a major driver of acute inflammation following lung contusion. Crit Care Med 2014;42(10):e642–53.
25. Beck-Schimmer B, Schimmer RC, Madjdpour C, et al. Hypoxia mediates increased neutrophil and macrophage adhesiveness to alveolar epithelial cells. Am J Respir Cell Mol Biol 2001;25(6):780–7 (In eng).
26. Suresh MV, Balijepalli S, Zhang B, et al. Hypoxia-Inducible Factor (HIF)-1alpha Promotes Inflammation and Injury Following Aspiration-Induced Lung Injury in Mice. Shock 2019;52(6):612–21.
27. Suresh MV, Balijepalli S, Zhang B, et al. Hypoxia-Inducible Factor (HIF)-1alpha Promotes Inflammation and Injury Following Aspiration-Induced Lung Injury in Mice. Shock 2018. https://doi.org/10.1097/SHK.0000000000001312.
28. Sturrock A, Woller D, Freeman A, et al. Consequences of Hypoxia for the Pulmonary Alveolar Epithelial Cell Innate Immune Response. J Immunol 2018;201(11):3411–20 (In eng).
29. Hanze J, Eul BG, Savai R, et al. RNA interference for HIF-1alpha inhibits its downstream signalling and affects cellular proliferation. Biochem Biophys Res Commun 2003;312(3):571–7.
30. Fish JE, Matouk CC, Yeboah E, et al. Hypoxia-inducible expression of a natural cis-antisense transcript inhibits endothelial nitric-oxide synthase. J Biol Chem 2007;282(21):15652–66.
31. Sun X, Kumar S, Sharma S, et al. Endothelin-1 induces a glycolytic switch in pulmonary arterial endothelial cells via the mitochondrial translocation of endothelial nitric oxide synthase. Am J Respir Cell Mol Biol 2014;50(6):1084–95.
32. Earley S, Resta TC. Estradiol attenuates hypoxia-induced pulmonary endothelin-1 gene expression. Am J Physiol Lung Cell Mol Physiol 2002;283(1):L86–93.
33. Pisarcik S, Maylor J, Lu W, et al. Activation of hypoxia-inducible factor-1 in pulmonary arterial smooth muscle cells by endothelin-1. Am J Physiol Lung Cell Mol Physiol 2013;304(8):L549–61.
34. Samanta D, Semenza GL. Maintenance of redox homeostasis by hypoxia-inducible factors. Redox Biol 2017;13:331–5.
35. Li Y, Jia A, Wang Y, et al. Immune effects of glycolysis or oxidative phosphorylation metabolic pathway in protecting against bacterial infection. J Cell Physiol 2019;234(11):20298–309 (In eng).
36. Semenza GL, Roth PH, Fang HM, et al. Transcriptional regulation of genes encoding glycolytic enzymes by hypoxia-inducible factor 1. J Biol Chem 1994;269(38):23757–63. Available at: https://www.ncbi.nlm.nih.gov/pubmed/8089148.
37. Semenza GL, Jiang BH, Leung SW, et al. Hypoxia response elements in the aldolase A, enolase 1, and lactate dehydrogenase A gene promoters contain essential binding sites for hypoxia-inducible factor 1. J Biol Chem 1996;271(51):32529–37.

38. Rodriguez-Prados JC, Traves PG, Cuenca J, et al. Substrate fate in activated macrophages: a comparison between innate, classic, and alternative activation. J Immunol 2010;185(1):605–14.

39. Kim JW, Tchernyshyov I, Semenza GL, et al. HIF-1-mediated expression of pyruvate dehydrogenase kinase: a metabolic switch required for cellular adaptation to hypoxia. Cell Metab 2006;3(3): 177–85.

40. Iyer NV, Kotch LE, Agani F, et al. Cellular and developmental control of O2 homeostasis by hypoxia-inducible factor 1 alpha. Genes Dev 1998;12(2): 149–62 (In eng).

41. Cheng SC, Quintin J, Cramer RA, et al. mTOR- and HIF-1alpha-mediated aerobic glycolysis as metabolic basis for trained immunity. Science 2014; 345(6204):1250684.

42. Eckle T, Brodsky K, Bonney M, et al. HIF1A reduces acute lung injury by optimizing carbohydrate metabolism in the alveolar epithelium. PLoS Biol 2013; 11(9):e1001665.

43. Selak MA, Armour SM, MacKenzie ED, et al. Succinate links TCA cycle dysfunction to oncogenesis by inhibiting HIF-alpha prolyl hydroxylase. Cancer Cell 2005;7(1):77–85.

44. D'Alessandro A, Moore HB, Moore EE, et al. Plasma succinate is a predictor of mortality in critically injured patients. J Trauma Acute Care Surg 2017;83(3):491–5.

45. Zhang H, Bosch-Marce M, Shimoda LA, et al. Mitochondrial autophagy is an HIF-1-dependent adaptive metabolic response to hypoxia. J Biol Chem 2008;283(16):10892–903 (In eng).

46. Zhang H, Gao P, Fukuda R, et al. HIF-1 inhibits mitochondrial biogenesis and cellular respiration in VHL-deficient renal cell carcinoma by repression of C-MYC activity. Cancer Cell 2007;11(5):407–20 (In eng).

47. Pak O, Scheibe S, Esfandiary A, et al. Impact of the mitochondria-targeted antioxidant MitoQ on hypoxia-induced pulmonary hypertension. Eur Respir J 2018. https://doi.org/10.1183/13993003. 01024-2017.

48. Meyrick B, Reid L. Endothelial and subintimal changes in rat hilar pulmonary artery during recovery from hypoxia. A quantitative ultrastructural study. Lab Invest 1980;42(6):603–15. Available at: https://www.ncbi.nlm.nih.gov/pubmed/6446620.

49. Stenmark KR, Meyrick B, Galie N, et al. Animal models of pulmonary arterial hypertension: the hope for etiological discovery and pharmacological cure. Am J Physiol Lung Cell Mol Physiol 2009; 297(6):L1013–32.

50. Forsythe JA, Jiang BH, Iyer NV, et al. Activation of vascular endothelial growth factor gene transcription by hypoxia-inducible factor 1. Mol Cell Biol 1996;16(9):4604–13.

51. Kouvaras E, Christoni Z, Siasios I, et al. Hypoxia-inducible factor 1-alpha and vascular endothelial growth factor in cartilage tumors. Biotech Histochem 2019;94(4):283–9.

52. Li J, Li SX, Gao XH, et al. HIF1A and VEGF regulate each other by competing endogenous RNA mechanism and involve in the pathogenesis of peritoneal fibrosis. Pathol Res Pract 2019;215(4):644–52.

53. Ceradini DJ, Kulkarni AR, Callaghan MJ, et al. Progenitor cell trafficking is regulated by hypoxic gradients through HIF-1 induction of SDF-1. Nat Med 2004;10(8):858–64.

54. Labrousse-Arias D, Castillo-Gonzalez R, Rogers NM, et al. HIF-2alpha-mediated induction of pulmonary thrombospondin-1 contributes to hypoxia-driven vascular remodelling and vasoconstriction. Cardiovasc Res 2016;109(1):115–30.

55. Gras E, Belaidi E, Briancon-Marjollet A, et al. Endothelin-1 mediates intermittent hypoxia-induced inflammatory vascular remodeling through HIF-1 activation. J Appl Physiol (1985) 2016;120(4):437–43.

56. Choi CW, Lee J, Lee HJ, et al. Deferoxamine Improves Alveolar and Pulmonary Vascular Development by Upregulating Hypoxia-inducible Factor-1alpha in a Rat Model of Bronchopulmonary Dysplasia. J Korean Med Sci 2015;30(9):1295–301.

57. Vadivel A, Alphonse RS, Etches N, et al. Hypoxia-inducible factors promote alveolar development and regeneration. Am J Respir Cell Mol Biol 2014; 50(1):96–105.

58. Tibboel J, Groenman FA, Selvaratnam J, et al. Hypoxia-inducible factor-1 stimulates postnatal lung development but does not prevent O2-induced alveolar injury. Am J Respir Cell Mol Biol 2015; 52(4):448–58.

59. Yu AY, Shimoda LA, Iyer NV, et al. Impaired physiological responses to chronic hypoxia in mice partially deficient for hypoxia-inducible factor 1alpha. J Clin Invest 1999;103(5):691–6.

60. Brusselmans K, Compernolle V, Tjwa M, et al. Heterozygous deficiency of hypoxia-inducible factor-2alpha protects mice against pulmonary hypertension and right ventricular dysfunction during prolonged hypoxia. J Clin Invest 2003;111(10):1519–27.

61. Steiner MK, Syrkina OL, Kolliputi N, et al. Interleukin-6 overexpression induces pulmonary hypertension. Circ Res 2009;104(2):236–44, 28p following 244.

62. Frid MG, Brunetti JA, Burke DL, et al. Hypoxia-induced pulmonary vascular remodeling requires recruitment of circulating mesenchymal precursors of a monocyte/macrophage lineage. Am J Pathol 2006;168(2):659–69.

63. Epelman S, Lavine KJ, Randolph GJ. Origin and functions of tissue macrophages. Immunity 2014; 41(1):21–35.

64. Leroyer AS, Blin MG, Bachelier R, et al. CD146 (Cluster of Differentiation 146). Arterioscler Thromb Vasc Biol 2019;39(6):1026–33.

65. Luo Y, Teng X, Zhang L, et al. CD146-HIF-1alpha hypoxic reprogramming drives vascular remodeling and pulmonary arterial hypertension. Nat Commun 2019;10(1):3551.

66. Tekin D, Dursun AD, Bastug M, et al. The effects of acute and intermittent hypoxia on the expressions of HIF-1alpha and VEGF in the left and right ventricles of the rabbit heart. Anadolu Kardiyol Derg 2011;11(5):379–85.

67. Liu W, Zhang Y, Lu L, et al. Expression and Correlation of Hypoxia-Inducible Factor-1alpha (HIF-1alpha) with Pulmonary Artery Remodeling and Right Ventricular Hypertrophy in Experimental Pulmonary Embolism. Med Sci Monit 2017;23:2083–8.

68. Tan Q, Kerestes H, Percy MJ, et al. Erythrocytosis and pulmonary hypertension in a mouse model of human HIF2A gain of function mutation. J Biol Chem 2013;288(24):17134–44.

69. Minamishima YA, Moslehi J, Bardeesy N, et al. Somatic inactivation of the PHD2 prolyl hydroxylase causes polycythemia and congestive heart failure. Blood 2008;111(6):3236–44.

70. Pullamsetti SS, Mamazhakypov A, Weissmann N, et al. Hypoxia-inducible factor signaling in pulmonary hypertension. J Clin Invest 2020;130(11):5638–51.

71. Bryant AJ, Carrick RP, McConaha ME, et al. Endothelial HIF signaling regulates pulmonary fibrosis-associated pulmonary hypertension. Am J Physiol Lung Cell Mol Physiol 2016;310(3):L249–62.

72. Fijalkowska I, Xu W, Comhair SA, et al. Hypoxia inducible-factor1alpha regulates the metabolic shift of pulmonary hypertensive endothelial cells. Am J Pathol 2010;176(3):1130–8.

73. Kurosawa R, Satoh K, Kikuchi N, et al. Identification of Celastramycin as a Novel Therapeutic Agent for Pulmonary Arterial Hypertension. Circ Res 2019;125(3):309–27.

74. Marsboom G, Toth PT, Ryan JJ, et al. Dynamin-related protein 1-mediated mitochondrial mitotic fission permits hyperproliferation of vascular smooth muscle cells and offers a novel therapeutic target in pulmonary hypertension. Circ Res 2012;110(11):1484–97.

75. Wilkins MR, Ghofrani HA, Weissmann N, et al. Pathophysiology and treatment of high-altitude pulmonary vascular disease. Circulation 2015;131(6):582–90.

76. Fu X, Zhang F. Role of the HIF-1 signaling pathway in chronic obstructive pulmonary disease. Exp Ther Med 2018;16(6):4553–61.

77. Aquino-Galvez A, Gonzalez-Avila G, Jimenez-Sanchez LL, et al. Dysregulated expression of hypoxia-inducible factors augments myofibroblasts differentiation in idiopathic pulmonary fibrosis. Respir Res 2019;20(1):130.

78. Bonnet S, Michelakis ED, Porter CJ, et al. An abnormal mitochondrial-hypoxia inducible factor-1alpha-Kv channel pathway disrupts oxygen sensing and triggers pulmonary arterial hypertension in fawn hooded rats: similarities to human pulmonary arterial hypertension. Circulation 2006;113(22):2630–41.

79. Dai Z, Li M, Wharton J, et al. Prolyl-4 Hydroxylase 2 (PHD2) Deficiency in Endothelial Cells and Hematopoietic Cells Induces Obliterative Vascular Remodeling and Severe Pulmonary Arterial Hypertension in Mice and Humans Through Hypoxia-Inducible Factor-2alpha. Circulation 2016;133(24):2447–58.

80. Wang M, Gu S, Liu Y, et al. miRNA-PDGFRB/HIF1A-lncRNA CTEPHA1 Network Plays Important Roles in the Mechanism of Chronic Thromboembolic Pulmonary Hypertension. Int Heart J 2019;60(4):924–37.

81. Han CF, Li ZY, Li TH. Roles of hypoxia-inducible factor-1alpha and its target genes in neonatal hypoxic pulmonary hypertension. Eur Rev Med Pharmacol Sci 2017;21(18):4167–80.https://www.ncbi.nlm.nih.gov/pubmed/29028080.

82. Lemus-Varela ML, Flores-Soto ME, Cervantes-Munguia R, et al. Expression of HIF-1 alpha, VEGF and EPO in peripheral blood from patients with two cardiac abnormalities associated with hypoxia. Clin Biochem 2010;43(3):234–9.

83. Farha S, Asosingh K, Xu W, et al. Hypoxia-inducible factors in human pulmonary arterial hypertension: a link to the intrinsic myeloid abnormalities. Blood 2011;117(13):3485–93.

84. Huang Y, Boerema-de Munck A, Buscop-van Kempen M, et al. Hypoxia inducible factor 2alpha (HIF2alpha/EPAS1) is associated with development of pulmonary hypertension in severe congenital diaphragmatic hernia patients. Pulm Circ 2018;8(3). 2045894018783734.

85. Tang H, Babicheva A, McDermott KM, et al. Endothelial HIF-2alpha contributes to severe pulmonary hypertension due to endothelial-to-mesenchymal transition. Am J Physiol Lung Cell Mol Physiol 2018;314(2):L256–75.

86. Marin-Hernandez A, Gallardo-Perez JC, Ralph SJ, et al. HIF-1alpha modulates energy metabolism in cancer cells by inducing over-expression of specific glycolytic isoforms. Mini Rev Med Chem 2009;9(9):1084–101.

87. Skuli N, Liu L, Runge A, et al. Endothelial deletion of hypoxia-inducible factor-2alpha (HIF-2alpha) alters vascular function and tumor angiogenesis. Blood 2009;114(2):469–77.

88. Zhang H, Qian DZ, Tan YS, et al. Digoxin and other cardiac glycosides inhibit HIF-1alpha synthesis and block tumor growth. Proc Natl Acad Sci U S A 2008;105(50):19579–86.

89. Abud EM, Maylor J, Undem C, et al. Digoxin inhibits development of hypoxic pulmonary hypertension in mice. Proc Natl Acad Sci U S A 2012;109(4):1239–44.

90. Dai Z, Zhu MM, Peng Y, et al. Therapeutic Targeting of Vascular Remodeling and Right Heart Failure in Pulmonary Arterial Hypertension with a HIF-2alpha Inhibitor. Am J Respir Crit Care Med 2018; 198(11):1423–34.

91. Hu CJ, Poth JM, Zhang H, et al. Suppression of HIF2 signalling attenuates the initiation of hypoxia-induced pulmonary hypertension. Eur Respir J 2019;54(6).

92. Wei H, Bedja D, Koitabashi N, et al. Endothelial expression of hypoxia-inducible factor 1 protects the murine heart and aorta from pressure overload by suppression of TGF-beta signaling. Proc Natl Acad Sci U S A 2012;109(14):E841–50.

93. Rosenkranz S, Feldman J, McLaughlin VV, et al. Selonsertib in adults with pulmonary arterial hypertension (ARROW): a randomised, double-blind, placebo-controlled, phase 2 trial. Lancet Respir Med 2022;10(1):35–46.